THE **IMPACT** OF **COLLECTIVE BARGAINING** ON **HOSPITALS**

THE IMPACT OF COLLECTIVE BARGAINING ON HOSPITALS

Richard U. Miller
Brian E. Becker
Edward B. Krinsky

PRAEGER

PRAEGER SPECIAL STUDIES • PRAEGER SCIENTIFIC

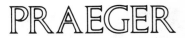

Library of Congress Cat .loging in Publication Data

Miller, Richard Ulric.
    The impact of collective bargaining on
hospitals.

    Bibliography: p.
    1. Collective bargaining--Hospitals--Illinois.
2. Collective bargaining--Hospitals--Minnesota.
3. Collective bargaining--Hospitals--Wisconsin.
I. Becker, Brian E., joint author. II. Krinsky,
Edward B., joint author. III. Title.
RA971.35.M55 331.89'041'362110977   79-9401
ISBN 0-03-051346-4

Published in 1979 by Praeger Publishers
A Division of Holt, Rinehart and Winston/CBS, Inc.
383 Madison Avenue, New York, New York 10017 U.S.A.

9 038 987654321

Printed in the United States of America

PREFACE AND
ACKNOWLEDGEMENTS

Industry studies of the influences of collective bargaining comprise a rich and varied literature in the fields of industrial relations and labor economics. Reflecting the ebb and flow of national policy issues, the focus of this line of research has moved from the manufacturing and extractive industries in the 1950s to the public sector in the 1970s. Continuing in this tradition, this study examines the impact of collective bargaining on an industry that has drawn a great deal of public attention in recent years and one that has been the focus of considerable attention by policy makers—the hospital industry.

Several characteristics of the recent history of the hospital industry make this research a timely effort. The tremendous growth in both the cost of hospital care and the level of employment in the industry underscore its growing importance to every aspect of the national economy. Within this setting, recent amendments to the National Labor Relations Act which extend bargaining rights to the employees of private, nonprofit hospitals raise the inevitable question of the effect of unionization on this critical industry. As labor costs represent nearly 60 percent of total costs in the industry, if unions have the same effect on wages and fringe benefits that have been reported for some of the manufacturing industries, the impact on hospital costs could be dramatic. Similarly, the specter of strikes and other job actions jeopardizing the quality of patient care has also been raised.

The purpose of this research is to offer some understanding of the nature and magnitude of these influences and replace at least some of this speculation with critical analysis. To accomplish this we have attempted to combine institutional and empirical methods of research so that they complement each other and enable us to pursue a broader range of union effects than are normally addressed in these studies.

The research reported here was initiated by means of a small award from the Graduate School of the University of Wisconsin, Madison, to study hospital labor relations in Wisconsin. Through a grant from the Labor Management Services Administration (LMSA) of the U.S. Department of Labor, the authors were able to expand the scope to include Minnesota and Illinois, in addition to Wisconsin.

The authors wish to express their appreciation to Herb Lahne, formerly of LMSA, who recognized the value of investigating healthcare labor relations, and to Leon Lunden of LMSA who, over many months, provided continuing support and encouragement.

64512

Many individuals and organizations assisted the investigators during the period of research. At the risk of failing to acknowledge important contributions, we would like to single out the following individuals who were helpful at various stages: Joseph Rosmann, American Hospital Association; Hervey Juris, Northwestern University; Don Wood and Earl Byrd, Chicago Hospital Council; John O'Donnell and Irving Perlmutter, Health Manpower Management, Inc. of Minneapolis-St. Paul; Warren Von Ehren, Wisconsin Hospital Association; Jim Pilz, Illinois Hospital Association; Lu Dewey Tanner, formerly of the Federal Mediation and Conciliation Service; Enid Weber, National Labor Relations Board; Morris Slavney, Wisconsin Employment Relations Commission; and Peter Verrochie, then with the U.S. Department of Labor.

The authors also wish to express their gratitude to Rudy Oswald, AFL-CIO; Don Wasserman, American Federation of State County and Municipal Employees; Neil Geske of Local 113 Service Employees International Union (SEIU); Irving Kurasch, Local 73, SEIU; June Watke, Wisconsin Nurses Association; Karen Patek, Minnesota Nurses Association; and Anne Zimmerman, Illinois Nurses Association.

The authors wish to acknowledge the important contribution of Norman Solomon of the Industrial Relations Research Institute, who was responsible for the Minnesota phase of the project and also assisted with the editing of the report in its many versions. A number of individuals also participated as project assistants in various phases of the study including, among others, Lee Running, Bette Briggs, Fred Burton, Joe Wiley, and Jack Bernfeld.

Finally, the authors owe a special sense of gratitude to Jeanne Meadowcraft and Linda Lucas. Jeanne Meadowcraft magically translated rough handwritten notes into earlier versions of this manuscript and proofread numerous drafts as well. Linda Lucas was responsible for the preparation and coordination of the final manuscript.

Neither the U.S. Department of Labor nor any of the individuals or organizations identified above is responsible for any misstatements or errors of fact contained in this book. All responsibility rests solely with the authors.

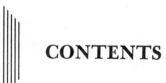

CONTENTS

LIST OF TABLES

1

INTRODUCTION

In the past two decades, the health-care industry has emerged as one of the major economic forces in the United States. Expenditures for health care now approach $163 billion, nearly 9 percent of the country's 1977 Gross National Product[1] and a tenfold increase over 1955 expenditures. In 1955 the proportion of the GNP accounted for by health-care expenditures was only 4.5 percent or $17 billion.

The explosive growth of expenditures for health care has been accompanied by an equally significant expansion in the number of persons working in the sector. In the 1960s, for example, employment rose by 65 percent, reaching 4.3 million in 1970.[2] This growth rate was three times greater than that of the economy as a whole. Although employment in the industry in the late 1970s may no longer be increasing as rapidly as earlier, the industry's rate of growth continues to exceed that of the labor force as a whole.[3]

Hospitals, the largest sector within the health-care industry, accounted for approximately 60 percent of the industry's employment in 1976 and for expenditures over $55 billion.[4] Moreover, annual surveys of the American Hospital Association (AHA) reveal that in each year since 1966, total hospital expenditures have increased 10 percent or more; in 1976 the increase was 14.3 percent.[5]

Governmental concerns with the cost of health care have led to numerous studies, hearings, and investigations, as well as wage and price controls between August 1971 and April 1974. Efforts to restrain these costs have met with little success as prices in this sector of the economy have continued to outstrip those in other sectors; in 1976, for example, the average cost of medical care rose twice as fast as the Consumer Price Index. By October 1978 the medical services price index for urban consumers had reached 241.8 in contrast to the CPI for all items, which measured 199.2 (CPI 1967 = 100.0).[6]

As might be expected, an important dimension of the economics of the health-care industry in general and hospitals in particular is the relationship of labor costs to total costs. In a labor-intensive industry, where payroll expenses accounted for 58 percent of total expenses in the average hospital in 1976,[7] the price of labor and the efficiency with which it is used obviously will have a major influence on the magnitude of health-care costs and the extent to which costs can be successfully controlled.

Given the above generalizations, it does not seem unreasonable to conclude that unions can have a significant impact on hospital costs and administrative control. One must then ask the empirical questions: What is the form of this impact, and how does it affect the cost and efficiency of the delivery of health care to the consumer?

Answers to such questions are partly contingent upon the incidence, strength, and militance of trade unions in the industry. As might be expected, given the late arrival of trade unionism to other service and professional occupations, collective bargaining is a recent phenomenon for health-care institutions. In 1967 only 7.7 percent of the hospitals in the United States had some form of labor agreement.[8] By 1975 this percentage had risen to 20.0 and can be expected to increase considerably beyond that figure by 1980.[9]

The rapid increase in unionization carried with it a by-product of conflict. During the decade of 1962-71, 248 strikes occurred, 50 percent of which grew out of demands for recognition.[10] One single strike in New York City involved 30,000 workers at 27 different hospitals. From January 1972 through December 1977, 337 work stoppages were recorded by the Bureau of Labor Statistics.[11] One is again confronted by such empirical questions as: How general are these strikes? Why do they occur? By what mechanisms do they get resolved?

RESEARCH OBJECTIVES

The literature describing labor-management relations in hospitals is inadequate for answering questions of the sort raised above,[†] and the published reports that do exist have been primarily case studies or speculative pieces based on anecdotal information. Thus, there is no firm basis in scientific and verifiable knowledge for the development of policy tools for dealing with the industry's labor problems.

[†]An attempt has been made in this study to identify and compile a bibliography of the most significant materials published since 1960.

We therefore sought to fill this gap through an intensive study of several aspects of hospital collective bargaining. The general goal was to gather and systematically analyze descriptive information about labor-management relations in the hospitals of three midwestern states: Illinois, Wisconsin, and Minnesota. In addition, three specific objectives within the general framework were selected: (1) to assess the impact of labor unions on wages, fringe benefits, and turnover, and the relation of these variables to overall hospital costs; (2) to evaluate the extent, if any, that contractual restrictions limit management's use of its hospital manpower; and (3) to identify the incidence, cause, and consequences of labor conflict in a hospital setting.

THE TRISTATE AREA OF ILLINOIS, MINNESOTA, AND WISCONSIN

The geographical scope of the research was limited to Illinois, Minnesota, and Wisconsin for several reasons. First, the development, history, and structure of hospital bargaining in the three states show great variation. As will be discussed in detail below, Minnesota constitutes one end of a spectrum with a high incidence of unionization, geographical diffusion, multiemployer bargaining units, and a low rate of conflict. At the opposite end is Illinois, exhibiting converse characteristics in nearly every respect. An intermediate position is appropriately occupied by Wisconsin, which shares certain collective bargaining characteristics with Illinois and others with Minnesota.

Second, the legal frameworks for trade unionism and collective bargaining in the three states differ. Until 1974, health-care institutions in Minnesota were covered by a special legislative enactment, the Charitable Hospitals Act (CHA). Wisconsin relied on a general labor law, the Wisconsin Employment Peace Act (WEPA), to handle health care as well as other industries over which the state had jurisdiction. On the other hand, Illinois had neither a labor law nor agencies; thus, the parties were forced to develop their own procedures.

Finally, the researchers had good contacts with and firsthand knowledge of the parties, so that the project could be formulated and carried out with the cooperation of the main practitioners of industrial relations in the three states. This cooperation was essential to the field interviews and mailed questionnaire survey that formed the main bases for data collection.

Thus, the tristate sample of hospitals provided sufficient variation to examine, on a cross-sectional basis, the differential impact on hospital bargaining of such institutional and organizational factors as legal framework, urban-rural location, size and mission of hospital, size of bargaining unit, and particular union involved.

Limiting the field of investigation to three states, while having obvious advantages, also has a major drawback that should be recognized at the outset. That is, the results reported here can be generalized to other sections of the United States or the country as a whole only with great caution. It is clear that the experience of the northeastern and Pacific Coast states, among others, has been quite different in many respects from that of our three midwestern states. At best, it is hoped that our conclusions may serve as reference points or hypotheses for others desiring to investigate hospital labor relations in other, perhaps broader, areas.

THE HOSPITAL AS A FOCUS FOR STUDY

Not only is our study limited geographically, but the research was intentionally further constrained by excluding all but short-term general-care community hospitals. Thus, unless otherwise stated, the following health-care institutions have been omitted: public and private nursing homes, governmentally owned and operated long-term hospitals, doctors' offices and clinics, and laboratories.

While it would have been interesting to study all health-care organizations, data collection would have been a major problem and the ability to make conclusions further impaired. However, over 85 percent of all hospitals in the three states are short-term, general-care hospitals, and they constitute the bulk of employing organizations in the health-care industry in the area and nationally. Further, they are reasonably homogeneous in character, with common organization and staffing patterns.

DATA AND SAMPLE

The data used in this study were developed from several sources. First, the American Hospital Association (AHA) Guide to Health Care Field was used to generate data on individual hospital size, expenses, services provided, and so forth.[†] A related AHA publication, Hospital Statistics, provided data on a national, state, and standard metropolitan statistical area (SMSA) basis.

[†]The Guide is published annually by the AHA and includes information on all member hospitals.

Another major source of area data was the U.S. Department of Health, Education, and Welfare publication <u>Hospitals: A County and Metropolitan Area Data Book</u>, [12] which includes 1970 census data on the number of hospitals, beds, and population by county. It was assumed that the counties are reasonably accurate proxies for local labor markets.

The primary source, however, was a mailed questionnaire sent to each of the 563 general-care, short-term hospitals in Illinois, Wisconsin, and Minnesota. (See Table 1.1.) The survey was designed to produce background information on each hospital and, more importantly, data on 12 occupations. [†] The occupations were selected on the basis of numerical importance in hospital operation, the likelihood that they might be covered by a collective bargaining agreement, and the ease with which the specific occupation could be communicated to the respondent (that is, a common occupation title used by most hospitals).

TABLE 1.1

Distribution of Questionnaire Responses

	Illinois (A)	Wisconsin (B)	Minnesota (C)	Total (D)
Total short-term, general-care hospitals in population	242	146	174	563
Percent of total	.43	.26	.31	1.00
Questionnaire response	63	40	41	144
Percent of total response	.44	.28	.28	1.00

Source: Compiled by the authors.

[†]The 12 occupations included staff pharmacist, physical therapist, general duty nurse, licensed practical nurse, nurse's aid, X-ray technologist, medical technologist, ward clerk, maid or porter, stationary engineer, kitchen helper, and switchboard operator.

The survey instrument was designed only after discussion with administrators in all three states. In addition, the questionnaire was pretested on a small sample of administrators in all three states, and the results were used to modify certain questions and reorganize the instrument.

Finally, it should be pointed out that numerous on-site interviews were conducted with union officials, hospital administrators, and third-party neutrals. With the assistance of such organizations as the American Hospital Association, the state hospital groups, and the Federal Mediation and Conciliation Service (FMCS) among others, institutional data were obtained by which the statistical analysis derived from the mailed questionnaire survey could be more fully interpreted. Particularly helpful in this regard were the interviews carried out in Chicago, Minneapolis-St. Paul, and Milwaukee.

ORGANIZATION

The remaining sections of this book will describe in detail the substance of the study and its findings. Chapter 2 provides an overview of the health-care industry in the three states, emphasizing trends in the industry, characteristics of employing institutions, and the structure and function of hospital labor markets. The legal framework for hospital labor relations in each of the three states is set out in detail in Chapter 3. Chapter 4 reviews the growth and extent of hospital unionism in each of the states, making public and private sector comparisons where feasible. The structure of collective bargaining in hospitals is considered in Chapter 5. Next, labor-management conflict, a major concern of all parties in the industry, is discussed in Chapter 6, where attention is given to the sources of conflict, the form in which conflict has emerged, and the use of different mechanisms for dispute resolution.

With the institutional framework thus established, the substantive issues that related directly to labor costs, compensation, and work force utilization are then subject to extensive analysis in Chapters 7 and 8. In Chapter 9, hospital-operating costs as they are affected by collective bargaining are examined. Finally, a summary and conclusions chapter attempts to integrate the different elements of hospital collective bargaining in Wisconsin, Illinois, and Minnesota, particularly with regard to implications for public policy.

NOTES

1. Robert M. Gibson and Charles R. Fisher, "National Health Expenditures, Fiscal Year 1977," Social Security Bulletin 41 (July 1978): 5.

2. Employment Impact of Health Policy Developments, National Commission for Manpower Policy, Special Report no. 11 (Washington, D.C.: 1976), p. 19.

3. Ibid.

4. Hospital Statistics (Chicago: American Hospital Association, 1977), p. v.

5. Ibid.

6. "The Consumer Price Index—October 1978," Bureau of Labor Statistics News (November 28, 1978), table 4.

7. Hospital Statistics, p. xvi.

8. "AHA Research Capsules—No. 6," Hospitals, JAHA 46 (April 1, 1972): 217.

9. Joseph Rossman, "One Year Under Taft-Hartley," Hospitals, JAHA 49 (December 16, 1975): 64.

10. U.S., Congress, Senate, Subcommittee on Labor of the Committee on Labor and Public Welfare, Hearings on S. 794 and S. 2292, 93rd Cong., 1st sess., July 31, August 1-2, and October 4, 1973, p. 243.

11. U.S., Department of Labor, Bureau of Labor Statistics, Division of Industrial Relations, personal communication to the authors.

12. U.S., Department of Health, Education, and Welfare, National Center for Health Statistics, Hospitals: A County and Metropolitan Area Data Book (Washington, D.C.: Government Printing Office, 1973).

2

THE HOSPITAL INDUSTRY: CHARACTERISTICS, TRENDS, AND PROBLEMS

NATIONAL DEVELOPMENTS

A recent publication recounting the history of hospital workers observes that "the early hospitals were not designed to treat the ill. They were places where the homeless and the poverty-stricken went to die. They were similar to alms-houses, institutions for people too poor to support themselves."[1] In fact, well into the twentieth century, hospitals were, as the Latin derivation implies, little more than hotels for the aged and acutely ill.

Technological change, scientific medicine, and miracle drugs produced a revolution in health care that continues. Thus, all phases of the modern hospital, from its mission to its architecture, have been revolutionized.[2] Automatic multiphasic laboratories, CAT body scanners, and organ transplants have become the hallmarks of the "health-care center" of the 1970s. Moreover, as John Knowles points out, good health is now considered a birthright, and Americans are demanding access to high-quality care.[3]

The transformation in the philosophy and practice of medicine is apparent in the manner in which the institutions that deliver health care themselves have changed. Thus, as Table 2.1 reveals, although the absolute numbers of hospitals have not changed, the jurisdictional control has shifted and, at the same time, gross assets have grown eight times since 1950. Public health care has shifted from federal to state and local government hospitals in a fashion paralleled by the decline of investor-owned or profit hospitals in favor of nongovernment, nonprofit institutions.

If one examines closely the trends in hospitals underlying the statistics presented in Table 2.1, the following picture emerges: (1) long-term stay hospitals (many of which are federal) are declining

8

TABLE 2.1

Hospitals in the United States

	Total	Federal	State and Local Government	Investor- Owned	Nongovernment Nonprofit	Total Assets (in millions)
1950	6,778	414	942	1,218	2,871	$7,791
1955	6,956	428	1,120	1,020	3,097	11,986
1960	6,876	435	1,260	856	3,291	17,714
1965	7,123	443	1,453	857	3,426	24,502
1970	7,123	408	1,704	769	3,386	36,159
1975	7,156	382	1,840	775	3,364	57,302
1976	7,082	308	1,836	752	3,368	64,029

Source: Hospital Statistics (Chicago: American Hospital Association, 1977), p. 3, table 1.

9

significantly; (2) short-term hospitals are not only increasing in importance, but are also undergoing important structural and administrative modifications; (3) the average number of beds per short-term community hospital is increasing (24 percent from 1965 to 1975); (4) the average rate of occupancy is down by 10 percent since 1950 and by nearly 8 percent since 1965; and (5) the number of out-patient visits is up by more than 100 percent since 1965 alone.[4]

In general, one can say that as hospital size increases, the likelihood that a hospital will offer a specialized service also rises.[5] This is particularly true of services that involve complex equipment, large capital investment, and more highly skilled personnel. Moreover, the ratio of full-time personnel is also positively correlated with the number of beds in a hospital. For example, AHA statistics indicate that hospitals with 24 or fewer beds averaged 1.7 full-time-equivalent personnel per bed while employing 36.5 percent part-time workers. For hospitals with 500 or more employees, the comparable figures were 3.1 full-time per bed and 15.7 percent part-time. As one might expect, the average salary of employees in such a hospital is 50 percent higher than that of their counterparts in the small hospitals.[6]

Given the demand for specialized services, difficulties in funding high-investment equipment, and soaring costs generally, the trend toward the large community hospital accelerated in the 1960s. As Table 2.2 demonstrates, large hospitals (400 or more beds) increased by 78 percent, moderate-sized hospitals (100-399 beds) by 24 percent, and those hospitals in the smallest categories (fewer than 100 beds) fell by 16 percent. As a consequence, the average community hospital in the United States had 163 beds in 1976, up from 129 eleven years earlier.

TABLE 2.2

Distribution of Community Hospitals by Number of Beds

Number of Beds	Number of Hospitals		Percent Change
	1965	1976	
6-24	562	290	-48.4
25-49	1,445	1,124	-22.2
50-99	1,482	1,446	-2.4
100-199	1,108	1,370	23.6
200-299	541	711	31.4
300-399	306	376	22.9
400-499	129	234	81.4
500 or more	163	306	87.7

Source: Hospital Statistics (Chicago: American Hospital Association, 1977), p. vii.

The movement toward larger hospitals and more specialized service in turn stimulated an increase in employment, particularly in the community hospitals. Thus, total hospital employment grew by 194 percent from 1950 to 1976 and by nearly 60 percent from 1965 to 1976. Over the same time periods, employment in short-term community hospitals grew 275 percent and 79 percent, respectively (see Table 2.3).

TABLE 2.3

Distribution of Full-Time-Equivalent Personnel in Hospitals
(in thousands)

| | Total U.S. | Federal | Short-Term Community | | |
			State and Local	Private Profit	Nongovernment Nonprofit
1950	1,058	169	148	41	473
1955	1,301	192	188	41	597
1960	1,598	186	241	48	792
1965	1,952	199	306	70	1,011
1970	2,537	216	444	97	1,387
1971	2,589	225	461	100	1,438
1972	2,671	232	477	105	1,474
1973	2,769	238	497	117	1,535
1974	2,919	244	522	133	1,634
1975	3,023	256	546	139	1,714
1976	3,108	269	543	147	1,793

Source: Hospital Statistics (Chicago: American Hospital Association, 1977), pp. 3-5.

Hospital financial structure and administration have also been revolutionized since 1950. The days when the average community hospital was dependent on charity for meeting its revenue shortfalls are long since gone. Equally vanished are the days when the health-care consumer paid the hospital directly. Public payment programs (Medicare, Medicaid, and MediCal, among others) and group health insurance, paid in part or completely by employers, have replaced historical systems of financing health-care expenditures.

In 1950, for example, consumers paid directly approximately two-thirds of the cost of their health care.[7] Public payments (22.4

percent) and insurance (9.1 percent) covered the remainder. By 1960, direct payments were 55 percent, with the remaining payments coming equally from public sources and insurance. As we might expect, particularly after the advent of Medicare and Medicaid in the mid-1960s, the shift accelerated in the source of funds for health-care expenditures so that by 1977 the consumer paid directly only 30 percent, insurance paid about 28 percent, and public payments exceeded 40 percent.[8] Third-party payments in 1977 constituted nearly 95 percent of hospital revenue.[9]

Moreover, the above figures may tend to understate the impact of the increasing incidence of insurance coverage on health-care delivery. Martin Feldstein estimates that over 95 percent of the American people are covered by some form of health insurance.[10] "Because hospital care is more completely insured than other health services, insurance distorts the pattern of health care toward the use of expensive hospital inpatient care . . .," "distorts the use of physicians services," and "distorts all aspects of patient care toward the increased use of services and toward the use of more expensive services."[11]

It is not surprising, therefore, that health-care expenditures and costs are rising rapidly. What is surprising is the magnitude of the increases and the apparent inability of the parties involved, short of complete price controls, to restrain these increases significantly. Thus, the President's Council on Wage and Price Stability reported in January 1977 that since 1950, in contrast to the general level of prices, which were up 125 percent, the cost of a day of hospital care rose by more than 1,000 percent.[12] Further, "the annual rate of increase in daily hospital costs accelerated sharply after 1966 when the Medicare and Medicaid programs were enacted."[13]

The rapid rise in health-care costs, the shift to public and insurance payments, and the precarious position of many community hospitals have inevitably led to outside intervention and control over hospital management. General rate review commissions have become commonplace in every state, public authorities have manipulated Medicare and Medicaid payments to force changes in hospital policies, and regional health-care planning bodies have sought to eliminate duplicate and excess facilities, to merge services, and, generally, to bring into better balance the allocation and distribution of health-care supply and demand. One of the most important steps in this direction was the advent of the concept of the "certificate of need" or "necessity" by which approval for the purchase of expensive equipment or new building construction would be granted only after extensive review by a designated public agency.

THE HOSPITAL INDUSTRY IN THE TRISTATE AREA

The generalizations made above for the most part are accurate also when applied to hospitals in Illinois, Minnesota, and Wisconsin. Thus, across the three states, hospitals tended to grow larger as measured by number of beds and, as a corollary, to offer more specialized services, employ more skilled workers, employ more workers per bed, pay higher salaries, and employ more full-time, as opposed to part-time, personnel. Moreover, short-term, public and nonprofit community hospitals have tended to displace long-term, either federal or investor-owned, health-care facilities.

Other characteristics that are also apparent at the regional level are declining occupancy rates, declining average length of stay, and increasing proportion of outpatient visits. These factors, when coupled with general inflation in the economy, produced the rise in health-care costs witnessed elsewhere in the country and triggered a concomitant intervention by public authorities.[14] Control by rate review boards or Medicare and Medicaid, however, had a less visible impact on the three states than was true of such regions as the Northeast. The prospect for such intervention, however, was growing, causing increasing controversy.[15]

An examination of the structure of the hospital industry in the three states suggests that the public and nonprofit, short-term community hospitals are the heart of the industry. In 1976, for the region as a whole, federal hospitals accounted for only approximately 3 percent of total hospitals, and those owned by private investors less than 2 percent (see Table 2.4). In addition, another 11 percent consisted of long-term state and private, nonprofit health-care facilities.

The three states individually reveal a number of interesting contrasts when data are disaggregated. For example, as Table 2.5 reveals, in Minnesota, small hospitals (6-99 beds) were the norm in 1976. In Wisconsin, hospitals were fairly evenly distributed between the small and intermediate-sized categories.

Illinois, with a population more than twice that of either of its sister states, not unexpectedly also had the largest hospital industry both in terms of absolute numbers of beds and personnel (see Table 2.6). By relative criteria, it was also the leader of the tristate area. That is, by such measures as beds per hospital, personnel per hospital, and personnel per bed, Illinois hospitals were larger by a significant amount. Moreover, this fact, when coupled with the greater number of personnel per bed, would suggest the availability of more specialized services. As indicated above, larger hospitals with more specialized services are associated with a higher proportion of full-time employees, higher skills, and, finally, higher salaries.

TABLE 2.4

Distribution of Hospitals and Personnel
in the Tristate Area, 1976

	Hospitals		Personnel	
Total	648	100.0%	306,158	100.0%
Private	420	64.8	220,695	72.1
Profit	8	1.2	867	*
Nonprofit	412	63.6	219,828	71.7
Public	155	23.9	54,600	28.0
State and local	137	21.8	36,621	12.0
Federal	18	2.8	17,974	5.9
Other	73	11.3	30,863	10.1

*Less than 1.0 percent.
Source: Hospital Statistics (Chicago: American Hospital
Association, 1977), table 5-C, pp. 66-67, 86-87, 138-39.

TABLE 2.5

Distribution of Hospitals by Number of Beds in Illinois,
Minnesota, Wisconsin, and the United States, 1976
(in percentages)

	Illinois	Minnesota	Wisconsin	U.S.
Small (6-99)	28.9	59.8	40.7	47.4
Intermediate (100-399)	50.9	26.5	49.4	39.7
Large (400 or more)	20.2	13.7	9.9	12.9

Source: Hospital Statistics (Chicago: American Hospital
Association, 1977), table 5-C, pp. 66-67, 86-87, 138-39.

TABLE 2.6

Distribution of Hospitals by Number of Beds and Personnel in
Illinois, Minnesota, Wisconsin, and the United States, 1976

	Illinois	Minnesota	Wisconsin	U.S.
Hospitals	287	189	172	7,082
Beds	77,312	31,385	31,146	1,433,515
Personnel	182,081	59,157	64,920	3,107,614
Beds/hospital	269	166	181	202
Personnel/hospital	634	313	377	438
Personnel/beds	2.3	1.9	2.1	2.2

Source: Hospital Statistics (Chicago: American Hospital
Association, 1977), table 5-C, pp. 66-67, 86-87, 138-39.

Minnesota's hospitals, smaller by half than those of Illinois,
had distinctly different characteristics from those of the other two
states. One would thus expect that these differences would be
paralleled by differences in the extent of unionism and the impact
of collective bargaining.

Wisconsin occupies a middle point on most measures of absolute and relative hospital size as depicted in Table 2.6. Consequently, at least as far as structural and administrative factors in hospitals affect unionization and collective bargaining in the industry,
Wisconsin should exhibit characteristics of both Illinois and Minnesota. We would hypothesize, however, based on Table 2.6, that to
the extent that characteristics differ, labor relations in Wisconsin
hospitals will more closely resemble those of Minnesota than Illinois.

NOTES

1. "Working in Hospitals: Then and Now," 1199 News, September 1976, p. 5.

2. John H. Knowles, "The Hospital," Scientific American,
September 1973, pp. 128-37.

3. Ibid., p. 130.

4. Hospital Statistics (Chicago: American Hospital Association, 1977), p. 3, table 1.

5. Ibid., p. xi.

6. Ibid., p. xiii.

7. Employment Impacts of Health Policy Developments, National Commission for Manpower Policy, Special Report no. 11 (1976), p. 34.

8. Robert M. Gibson and Charles R. Fisher, "National Health Expenditures, Fiscal Year 1977," Social Security Bulletin 41 (July 1978): 7.

9. Ibid.

10. Martin Feldstein, "The Medical Economy," Scientific American, September 1973), p. 155.

11. Ibid., pp. 151-53.

12. Martin Feldstein and Amy K. Taylor, The Rapid Rise of Hospital Costs (Washington, D.C.: Council on Wage and Price Stability, 1977), p. ii.

13. Ibid.

14. For example, see "[Governor] Lucey Asks Health Reins," Wisconsin State Journal, March 20, 1977.

15. Reid Beveridge, "Health Facilities Restrictions Get Cold Reception at Meet," Wisconsin State Journal, February 24, 1977.

3

THE LEGAL FRAMEWORK FOR HOSPITAL LABOR RELATIONS IN ILLINOIS, WISCONSIN, AND MINNESOTA

Hospitals do not exist in isolation from the economic, social, and legal systems that surround them. Thus, such questions as whether smaller hospitals are more prone to unionization, whether collective bargaining increases labor costs or work force misallocation, and whether traditional mechanisms of labor dispute resolution are successful in a hospital setting can be answered only by reference to the relevant contexts within which the industrial relations systems operate.[1]

This chapter will examine one of the major environmental influences on labor relations, the legal framework for collective bargaining. The legal frameworks of the three states, characterized by great diversity before the advent of the health-care amendments to the Taft-Hartley Act, had important implications for the extent of unionization, the structure of collective bargaining, and the incidence of labor conflict. Moreover, the existing framework influenced the effectiveness of the federal law after 1974.

PRE-1974 LEGAL FRAMEWORK

The enactment, in August 1974, of the health-care amendments to the Taft-Hartley Act is an appropriate line of demarcation for purposes of analyzing the legal framework for bargaining in hospitals. Before 1974, private, nonprofit hospitals were subject to a diverse collection of state jurisdictions, many of which, either by explicit prohibition or implicitly through their silence on the subject, constituted an obstacle not only to collective bargaining but to unionization as well. Those states that did provide for specific control over hospital labor relations created a legacy that has

17

carried over into the period of federal regulation. Thus, while in theory a unified and standardized public policy has existed since 1974, many previously established hospital bargaining relationships still reflect the earlier state control.

Illinois

Like 38 other states in this category, Illinois provided no regulation of bargaining in the nonprofit health-care sector by statute or agency. As a consequence, "nonprofit hospitals [were] in no way required to recognize or bargain collectively with their employees."[2]

Illinois, however, did possess a "mini" Norris-LaGuardia or Anti-Injunction Act,[3] which was applied to nonprofit hospitals. Thus, the Illinois Supreme Court ruled in 1969 that "the language of the statute is clear, and it makes no exception for hospitals."[4] In observing that "this is the only legislative expression of public policy which touches on the labor relations of these not-for-profit hospitals," the court admonished the legislature to take action for this sector beyond what was expressed in the Anti-Injunction Act.[5] The Illinois legislature, for whatever reason, declined to act on the court's suggestion.

With no mechanisms for dispute settlement and given total freedom to use whatever power could be exerted, it is not surprising that a significant characteristic of health-care labor relations in Illinois was open conflict. If a union was to achieve even minimal recognition, a work stoppage was necessary. Thus, from 1966 when union organizing began in earnest through 1974 when federal jurisdiction was established, Illinois had 13 private sector hospital strikes; Wisconsin had four, and there were none in Minnesota.[6]

In the public sector, the picture is even more graphic, showing a record 25 strikes in governmental hospitals in Illinois over the same time period. Wisconsin and Minnesota, each with extensive labor legislation covering both public and private sectors, experienced five strikes and no strikes, respectively.[7] The work stoppages occurred in the Illinois public sector despite the apparent illegality of concerted action by public employees.[8]

The lack of a legislated framework for bargaining in Illinois not only resulted in a great deal of labor conflict, but also forced the parties to attempt to create their own mechanisms for handling recognition and negotiation disputes. Thus, for example, in the Chicago area the major labor union active in the hospital industry, the Health Employees Labor Program (HELP), attempted to persuade the Illinois court to require representation elections and a

duty to bargain with elected representatives of hospital employees.
When this tactic was unsuccessful, HELP turned to negotiating
election agreements directly with the hospitals.[9] The procedure,
used in more than 31 elections through 1974, provided for an election to be held, a one-year ban on future organizing if HELP lost,
a no-strike-no-lockout agreement, and arbitration of grievance and
negotiation impasses.[†]

Preelection consent agreements were not always agreed to
voluntarily. For example, in the case of Walther Memorial Hospital
in Chicago, the agreement to hold an election came only after a
17-day strike. In the case of the South Chicago Community Hospital,
a strike for such ends was unsuccessful. Thus, until the federal
law took effect, hospital labor and management in Illinois used
whatever means at their disposal to persuade—or compel—the
opposing party to concede in recognition and contract disputes.

Wisconsin

The legal framework for hospital collective bargaining in
Wisconsin stands in stark contrast to that of Illinois. The general
state labor code from 1943 on provided hospital employees and
management with access to the Wisconsin Employment Relations
Commission (WERC) in cases of disputes over recognition and
unfair labor practices, and for mediation of contract (interest) disputes.[10] The Wisconsin Employment Peace Act made no distinction
between private, nonprofit hospitals and other private employers in
the state. Consequently, hospital management was free to lock out,
and hospital employees were free to engage in work stoppages without constraints or conditions. The WEPA apparently was unique in
this respect among state statutes.[11]

Public hospital employees in Wisconsin are covered under
specific state laws, depending on the political authority having jurisdiction over the hospital. For example, county and municipal health-
care organizations are subject to the Municipal Employment Relations Act (MERA) of 1959.[12] For those workers employed by the
state, the appropriate statute is the State Employment Labor Relations Act (SELRA), enacted in 1972.[13] SELRA and MERA were

---

[†]Depending on the agreement, elections were supervised by one
of the following three parties: the Illinois State Department of Labor,
the American Arbitration Association, or Ann Miller, a private attorney in Chicago.

quite consistent with the general labor code in all respects save one—
an outright prohibition on strikes, with various penalties provided in
the event of violation. Moreover, the statutes also prescribed mediation and nonbinding fact finding in those cases involving disputes
over contract negotiations. In November 1977, the Municipal Employment Relations Act was amended to provide for a limited right
to strike as an option to binding arbitration of new contract disputes.

Minnesota

The labor statutes that covered Minnesota hospital employees
prior to 1974 provide a second contrast to those of Illinois. In the
period 1939 to 1947, hospital workers were covered by the Minnesota Labor Relations Act, a little Wagner Act, and recognition and
other disputes were handled by the state's labor board, the Bureau
of Mediation Services. In this early period, hospitals were treated
no differently from other employers with the result that strikes,
picketing, and lockouts were legal.

The state legislature, however, enacted the Charitable Hospitals Act (CHA) in 1947 as an amendment to the general labor code.
The CHA was a response to actual or threatened strikes by hospital
employees and forbade all health-care work stoppages, whether in
the public or private sectors.[14]

Although bitterly opposed by labor organizations, the act was
held constitutional by the Minnesota Supreme Court in 1954 as a
legitimate exercise of the state's police power.[15] In the same case,
the court interpreted the Charitable Hospitals Act's stated applicabil-
ity to "any unsettled issues of maximum hours of work and minimum
hourly wage" as including economic and welfare matters except
those associated with the union shop, union security, or "the internal
management of such hospitals."[16]

The success of the CHA in avoiding labor strife in the hospital
industry of Minnesota can be seen from statistics on work stoppages.
Over the years since its enactment, only one strike occurred, and
that a brief one; since 1965, no work stoppages of record took place.

The success of the Charitable Hospitals Act led New York
State to use it as a model in drafting similar statutes beginning in
1963.[17] A point of difference between the New York version and
Minnesota's CHA was that in the latter law arbitration could be re-
quested only by labor or management, or both. New York stipulated
that the state also could initiate arbitration. It is of interest to note
that hospital strikes continued unabated in New York after its law
was passed, and virtually no effort was made by the state to compel
use of the dispute settlement procedures.

An additional measure of the acceptance of the CHA in Minnesota emerged when the federal law became effective. With the concurrence of the parties, the state petitioned the National Labor Relations Board (NLRB) on March 10, 1975, to cede jurisdiction of health-care cases to Minnesota. The board, in a unanimous decision handed down August 15, 1975, denied the petition.[18] In rejecting Minnesota's request, the board cited the fact that Minnesota's CHA was in conflict with federal law at three points: the right to strike and the right to lock out, both permitted under federal law, and the use of compulsory arbitration, which federal law does not require.

Following rejection of the petition, the parties to a number of major hospital contracts in Minnesota voluntarily agreed to settle negotiating impasses through binding arbitration for periods up to ten years. Thus, while the New York State version of the CHA may have been perceived as unworkable, the parties in Minnesota obviously did not share that conviction.

POST-1974 LEGAL FRAMEWORK

The adoption of the 1974 health-care amendments was preceded by a long and sometimes bitter struggle by labor organizations to rescind the nonprofit hospital exemption to federal labor law protection that had been placed in the National Labor Relations Act in 1947. Prior to the passage of the Taft-Hartley Act, federal law made no specific mention of hospitals; therefore, it was left to the NLRB and the courts to decide what had been the intent of Congress when the original law was enacted in 1935.

With no legislative standards for bench marks, the intent of Congress was generally perceived to be that private hospitals were not excluded from the law's coverage.[19] However, since such hospitals were deemed charitable, nonprofit institutions not motivated by monetary considerations, the board concluded that it was not in the public interest to assert jurisdiction over them.

In view of the foregoing, the inclusion of a specific exemption for private, nonprofit hospitals from the federal labor code in 1947 was not surprising. One could reasonably conclude that this was merely a reflection of general community values. In fact, the major arguments for an exclusion put forth at the hearings on the Senate floor by Senator Tydings said as much.

> This amendment is designed merely to help a great
> number of hospitals which are having very difficult
> times. They are eleemosynary institutions; no

> profit is involved in their operation; and I understand
> from the Hospital Association that this amendment
> would be very helpful in their efforts to serve those
> who have not the means to pay for hospital service,
> enable them to keep their doors open, and operate
> the hospitals.[20]

There was little debate on this point. Thus, in its final version, the Taft-Hartley Act carried, in its section 2(2) definition of employer, the exemption of "any corporation or association operating a hospital, if no part of the net earnings insures to the benefit of any private shareholder or individual."[21] For 12 years thereafter, the major component of the health-care industry in the United States, 4,000 hospitals with 1.6 million workers, was left to the vagaries of state common or statutory labor law.

Other segments of the industry, however, slowly became subject to federal rules. Among the first were the federal hospitals, which came under the Executive Orders of Presidents Kennedy (10988) and Nixon (11491) issued in 1962 and 1970, respectively. In addition, although the section 2(2) definition of employers excluded private, nonprofit hospitals, it seemed to leave the door open to coverage of investor-owned hospitals and private nursing homes whether operated for profit or not. Thus, the NLRB gradually began to expand its health-care jurisdiction beginning with proprietary hospitals (1967),[22] nursing homes (1967),[23] and nonprofit nursing homes (1970).[24]

By the early 1970s, the validity of the premises upon which the 2(2) exemption was based came under increasing attack from industry representatives as well as those of labor. Most notable among them was Norman Metzger, breaking ranks with his management colleagues, who argued:

> It was incomprehensible that an industry as large, as
> complex, as interstate in nature and as important as
> [health care], should today be excluded from the national labor laws. It is essential, to end the chaos
> and inequities that presently exist in nonprofit hospital
> labor relations and to avoid future chaos and inequities,
> that the exemption of nonprofit hospitals from the provisions of the National Labor Relations Act be rescinded
> at the earliest possible moment.[25]

After an aborted attempt in 1971, a second effort to remove the 2(2) exemption succeeded, resulting in the enactment of P.L. 93-360 on July 26, 1974. What so long had eluded the labor organizations in health care seemed to have been achieved: the states were now preempted from asserting jurisdiction over nonprofit hospitals, and the federal government apparently had endorsed collective bargaining for the industry.

P. L. 93-360

The 1974 amendments not only deleted nonprofit hospitals from the employer exemption of Section 2(2) of the Taft-Hartley Act, but also introduced several new legal conditions that would be unique to hospitals:

(1) Notice of intent to strike or picket must be made ten days before such action takes place.

(2) Notification of intent to modify or terminate existing contracts is to be made by the parties 90 days beforehand; the Federal Mediation and Conciliation Service is to be notified 60 days in advance. The like requirement for other industries continues at 60 and 30 days, respectively.

(3) The parties are required to participate in mediation efforts offered by the FMCS in the event of a dispute.

(4) Boards of inquiry (BOIs) are to be established if, in the opinion of the director of FMCS, a strike or lockout will "substantially interrupt the delivery of health care in the locality concerned." The BOI must be set up within 30 days after the Conciliation Service is notified by the parties of an impending dispute (as required by the 90 and 60 day notification section of the law) and 15 days before the final notification period expired, the BOI would issue its nonbinding report.

(5) Members of religious sects are exempted from union security provisions, but must pay the equivalent in union dues or fees to charitable organizations specified by the parties in the contract.

(6) The NLRB must avoid "proliferation of bargaining units in health care institutions."[26]

The amendments extend to all private, profit, and nonprofit health-care employees the right to engage in strikes, picketing, and other forms of concerted activity. Congress's concern with minimizing disruptions in the delivery of health care when these rights are exercised is reflected throughout the amendments. Thus, the stipulation that parties will notify each other 90 days before modification of existing contracts makes it an unfair labor practice to strike during this period. Further, mediation is mandatory following the 60-day notice to FMCS of intent to terminate or modify a contract. In addition, the condition of a ten-day notice before either a strike or picketing commences would enable the health institutions involved to make preparations to transfer or otherwise ensure the safety of patients. In this respect also, the "ally doctrine" would not be applied to hospitals receiving patients from threatened or struck institutions.

Although Congress stopped short of requiring compulsory binding arbitration, it did insert through the boards of inquiry a fact-finding step that could be invoked at the discretion of the FMCS.

P.L. 93-360 in Retrospect

It would be surprising if, in the years since their passage, all parties in health-care bargaining—labor, management, government—were satisfied with the 1974 amendments. As might be expected, all parties are not satisfied, for some very predictable reasons.

A great deal of contention centers on the hospital bargaining units drawn up by the NLRB. Beginning with a series of eight decisions handed down in May 1975, the board has decreed that there are to be five basic units: (1) registered nurses (RNs), (2) other health-care professionals, (3) technical employees, (4) service and maintenance employees, and (5) business office clericals.[27] A sixth unit, employee physicians, was added in July 1977.[28]

For the International Union of Operating Engineers (IUOE) and similar labor organizations, the decisions seemed to signal the end of a separate bargaining unit for stationary engineers and maintenance workers in hospitals. Other unions such as District 1199,[†] the Service Employees International Union (SEIU), and the Retail Clerks International Association (RCIA), initially greeted service and maintenance units enthusiastically.

The professional employees and their organizations viewed the technical unit with mixed emotions. For the licensed practical nurses (LPNs), it was a mark of reduced professional status to be

---

[†]Formally known as National Union of Hospital and Health Care Employees, a division of the Retail, Wholesale, and Department Store Union (RWDSU), AFL-CIO.

excluded from the bargaining unit of the registered nurses. Some
members of other occupational groups would be placed in the technical unit and some in the professional unit. The board, in differen-
tiating between the two groups, concluded that in addition to being
licensed or certified, an employee must hold a minimum of a
baccalaureate degree to be considered a professional.

For the numerous hospital professionals such as pharmacists,
occupational therapists, physical therapists, and allied employees,
the general professional unit signified a loss of autonomy and a
potential loss of identity. These employees felt no community of
interest with each other and had no natural organization around
which to group for representational and bargaining purposes. In
their view, assignment to the general professional unit would be a
step backward.

Hospital management, on the other hand, shared the general
negative reaction to the board's unit decisions, favoring much
broader bargaining units. Foreseeing the possibility of as many as
11 or 12 units, hospital representatives contended, "The board has
permitted unit proliferation in hospitals."[29] The board's unit policy
was decried as inconsistent with the mandate placed by Congress on
the NLRB when the amendments were enacted.

Industry representatives felt that separate units of nurses
were not justifiable, nor did they accept units for technical employees different from those in service and maintenance categories.[30]
Reluctant applause was given, however, to the NLRB's policy of rejecting distinct maintenance units, although it was coupled with
apprehension that the board was not holding firm to this policy at all
times.[31]

Perhaps the major criticism of board unit policy arose in connection with its decision that hospital residents and interns (housestaff) did not meet the act's definition of employee.[32] This decision,
together with a later one by the NLRB that, notwithstanding the exclusion from the employee definition, federal law preempted states
from acting, left the residents and interns in a legal "no-man's-
land."[33] The lack of federal labor law protections for housestaff
organizations has made it possible for hospitals to refuse to recognize and bargain with residents and interns.

The NLRB's position on this issue provoked dissension within
itself[34] and another effort in Congress to overrule the board's
policy by amending the law.† Although the bill was opposed by the

---

†On January 19, 1977, H.R. 2222 was introduced in the House
by Chairman Frank Thompson of the House Subcommittee on Labor.

American Hospital Association, notable supporters included the American Medical Association.[35]

Other board policies that came under fire were its handling of issues involving registered nurses as supervisors, the extent to which professional associations such as the American Nurses Association constitute legally defined labor organizations, and what are perceived to be general delays in processing election petitions and unfair labor practice complaints.[36]

The NLRB thus was a focal point for controversy over the 1974 amendments. Sharing this criticism, however, was the Federal Mediation and Conciliation Service that was given the duty under P. L. 93-360 to administer the notification, mediation, and boards of inquiry changes in the law. Labor organizations complained that BOIs were appointed too infrequently, both labor and management were critical of the quality of persons appointed to the BOIs, and various groups including the FMCS cited the time periods for the BOIs' appointment and report as unrealistic.[37]

IMPACT OF P. L. 93-360 ON HEALTH-CARE LABOR
RELATIONS IN THE TRISTATE AREA

Although at this writing it is still early to reach firm conclusions, the effect of the 1974 amendments in the tristate area appears at best neutral and in some cases negative. In Illinois, the high incidence of hospital conflict does not appear to have diminished. Despite this, the FMCS has chosen not to use the BOI procedure; it was invoked in only one case between 1974 and 1977.

In addition, labor organizations in Illinois are quick to point out that even though no statutory collective bargaining rights existed under state law, there were also no constraints on the use of collective action. If recognition was not granted, the union was free to strike, picket, or use whatever force was available, which led ultimately and frequently to preelection agreements and informal systems of dispute resolution.

In Minnesota and Wisconsin, federal law preempted state laws that already provided rights and protections as well as machinery for handling recognition and bargaining disputes. As far as labor was concerned, the amendments conferred a series of dubious benefits: the right to strike, which Wisconsin already had and which unions in Minnesota were quite willing to bargain away; access to the NLRB whose administrative apparatus seemed to operate at a much slower pace than that of the state labor boards; and an NLRB bargaining unit policy whose representation election boundaries tended to be much broader than those permitted by the states. The unions were convinced that smaller units were easier to organize and consequently groups such as pharmacists or skilled maintenance people could be "appropriately" represented. Furthermore, elections were not stalled over endless "employer-inspired" delays.

The long-awaited incorporation of nonprofit hospitals into the federal labor law did not produce a massive and rapid unionization of hospitals in the three states. The results of more than four years of union efforts to organize health-care institutions in Illinois, Minnesota, and Wisconsin seem to support the conclusion that, at least in 1978, the collective bargaining benefits of the 1974 amendments were still to be realized.

NOTES

1. On this point, see John Dunlop, Industrial Relations Systems (New York: Henry Holt, 1958), p. 9.

2. Norman Metzger and Dennis W. Pointer, Labor Management Relations in the Health Services Industry: Theory and Practice (Washington: Science and Health, 1972), p. 63.

3. Illinois Revised Statutes, ch. 48, sec. 2(a), amended 1973.

4. Peters v. South Chicago Community Hospital, 44 Ill. 2d 22, 253 N.E. 2d 375 (1969).

5. Ibid.

6. Bureau of Labor Statistics, Work Stoppages Section, personal communication to the authors, April 15, 1977.

7. Ibid.

8. Board of Education v. Redding, 32 Ill. 2d 567, 207 N.E. 2d 427 (1965); and County of Peoria v. Benedict, 47 Ill. 2d 166, 265 N.E. 2d 141 (1970).

9. Ronald L. Miller, "Collective Bargaining in Non-Profit Hospitals," (Ph.D. diss., University of Pennsylvania, 1969), pp. 274-77.

10. Wisconsin Employment Peace Act, WS111. 01-111.17, Laws of Wisconsin 1939, as amended by ch. 245; 1. 1971.

11. Miller, "Collective Bargaining," pp. 254-55.

12. WS 111.70-111.77. Laws of Wisconsin 1959 as amended by ch. 247; 1. 1971 and 1977.

13. WS 111.80-111.97. Laws of Wisconsin 1971.

14. Miller, "Collective Bargaining," p. 233.

15. Fairview Hospital Association v. Public Building Service Union, 241 Minn. 523, 64 N.W. 2d 16 (1954).

16. Ibid.

17. Miller, "Collective Bargaining," p. 240; see also Metzger and Pointer, Labor Management Relations, p. 65.

18. Office of the General Council, NLRB, Press Release (August 15, 1975).

19. Central Dispensary and Emergency Hospital v. NLRB, 145 F.2d 852 (D.C. Cir. 1944), cert. denied 324 U.S. 827 (1944).

20. Congressional Record, 93, 1947, pt. 4: 4997.

21. Labor Management Relations Act, Public Law 101, 80th Cong., 1st sess., 1947.

22. Butte Medical Properties, 168 NLRB 266 (1967).

23. University Nursing Home, Inc., 168 NLRB 53 (1967).

24. Drexel Homes, 194 NLRB 63 (1970).

25. U.S., Congress, House, Special Subcommittee on Labor of the Committee on Education and Labor, Extension of NLRA to Nonprofit Hospital Employees, Hearings on H.R. 11357, 92d Cong., 1st and 2d sess., 1972, p. 173. See also, Dennis D. Pointer and Norman Metzger, The National Labor Relations Act: A Guidebook for Health Care Facility Administrators (New York: Spectrum, 1975), pp. 41-55.

26. See Pointer and Metzger, National Labor Relations Act, pp. 55-60.

27. Mercy Hospitals of Sacramento, Inc., 217 NLRB 131 (1975); Barnert Memorial Hospital Association, 217 NLRB 132 (1975); St. Catherine's Hospital of Dominican Sisters, 217 NLRB 133 (1975); Newington Children's Hospital, 217 NLRB 134 (1975); Sisters of St. Joseph of Peace, 217 NLRB 135 (1975); Duke University, 217 NLRB 136 (1975); Mount Airy Foundation, 217 NLRB 137 (1975); and Shriners Hospital for Crippled Children, 217 NLRB 138 (1975).

28. Ohio Valley Hospital Association, 230 NLRB 84 (1977).

29. See the remarks of William Emanuel as reported in Bureau of National Affairs, Daily Labor Report, no. 86 (May 3, 1977), p. A12.

30. Ibid.

31. Analysis of NLRB representation election results indicate that nearly 60 craft unit elections were held in hospitals over the period August 1974 through August 1978. The majority (37) were on the initiative of the Operating Engineers Union. Criticism of its decision of designating separate bargaining units for maintenance or power plant employees finally elicited a strong disclaimer by the board in December 1978. See Allegheny General Hospital 239 NLRB 104 (1978).

32. Cedars-Sinai Medical Center, 223 NLRB 57 (1976).

33. Kansas General Hospital, 225 NLRB 14 (1976); but also see NLRB v. Committee of Interns and Residents et al., U.S. District Court of Southern New York, case No. 76 Cov. 5119, January 31, 1977.

34. Bureau of National Affairs, Daily Labor Report, no. 86 (May 3, 1977), p. D3. At the American Bar Association's April 28, 1977 National Institute on Hospitals and Health Care Facilities, newly appointed chairman of the NLRB, John H. Fanning, stated: "No matter how viable, in a vacuum, the arguments may be for excluding doctors from coverage (and no one disputes that housestaff are doctors), from the standpoint of the fundamental purposes of the statute and amendments, the very reason for their existence, the exclusion of housestaff is, in my view, untenable." See also Fanning's dissent in the Cedars-Sinai decision.

35. Bureau of National Affairs, Daily Labor Report, no. 65 (April 4, 1977), p. A13.

36. See Bureau of National Affairs, White Collar Report, no. 976 (December 19, 1975), p. A2. The NLRB has been described by some labor leaders as "the graveyard for union aspirations." At the Second Biennial Convention of the National Union of Hospital and Health Care Employees (District 1199 of RWDSU), Leon Davis, the union's president, commented that he expected hostility from hospital management but "did not anticipate the obstruction of the National Labor Relations Board." He was quoted further as saying: "This Board has supersensitive ears and sympathy for management but turns a deaf ear to workers. [Management's] sabotage of the Act takes on the form of endless hearings and interminable delays, so that the workers become frustrated, and management takes advantage of these delays by conducting anti-union campaigns and destroying the will of the workers for a union. Even if the union wins, the Board has no power or will to compel management to bargain collectively in good faith or to sign a contract with the union."

37. See the comments of Herb Fishgold, General Counsel for FMCS and Nicholas Fidandis, also of FMCS, in Bureau of National Affairs, Daily Labor Report, no. 86 (May 3, 1977), pp. A14-A17.

4

THE INCIDENCE OF
HOSPITAL UNIONISM

Not very many years ago, the health care industry was clearly
virgin territory for unions. As Table 4.1 reveals, barely 3 percent
of the hospitals in the United States had contracts with labor organizations in 1961. Public hospital employees were virtually without
union representation. By 1967, this situation was beginning to change
significantly, particularly in federal hospitals where Kennedy's Executive Order 19088 stimulated organization.

TABLE 4.1

Percentage of Hospitals with One or More Union Contracts

	Total	Federal	State and Local Government	Private Nonprofit	Investor- Owned Profit
1975	19.8	75.4	19.0	16.9	9.8
1973	16.8	63.2	16.6	13.9	8.0
1970	14.7	52.0	14.1	12.4	8.0
1967	7.7	22.6	5.3	8.2	4.9
1961	3.0	0.0	1.0	4.3	4.3

Sources: 1961-70: "AHA Research Capsules—No. 6," Hospitals, JAHA 46 (April 1, 1972): 217. 1973-75: Personal communication to the authors from the Employee Relations and Training Department, American Hospital Association.

The growth of unionization continued into the decade of the 1970s to such an extent that by 1977 nearly one in every five hospitals was unionized. The leading edge of unionizing continued to be in the public sector, especially in the federal hospitals.

The distribution of hospitals with union contracts in the private sector indicates a number of interesting contrasts. On the one hand, despite the fact that investor-owned hospitals have been covered by federal law since 1967, they show a significantly lower proportion of union contracts. In addition (not shown in Table 4.1), church-affiliated hospitals have the lowest rate of union contracts of any health-care institutions in either the private or public sector, barely exceeding 1 percent in 1975.[1]

Regionally, hospital unionism tends to be concentrated in the Northeast (New York, Connecticut, and Massachusetts), the Pacific Coast (California, Oregon, and Washington), and the Midwest (Minnesota and Michigan).[2] Interestingly enough, the state with the highest proportion of hospitals under union contract is Hawaii (nearly 90 percent).

The fact that across the hospital industry only 20 percent of hospital employees are covered by union contracts indicates that this industry is only slightly less a union "no-man's-land" in 1978 than it was in the early 1960s.[3] Despite indications that, in the aftermath of the changes in the federal law, unions were significantly increasing both their organizing activity and their election success,[4] the early pace apparently has not continued. For example, the proportion of elections won by unions was higher than the general industry rate from August 1974 to July 1975, namely, 56 percent as opposed to 50 percent. In the second year (1975-76), the proportion of wins dropped to slightly over 50 percent. By January 1978 the ratio of representation victories to losses had fallen further to 45.8 percent.[5]

If it is assumed that the most vulnerable hospitals were organized in the months immediately after the passage of the health-care amendments, the proportion of wins to losses was bound to decline. Further, hospital managements increasingly resorted to outside consultants to counter union-organizing drives. Where consultants were used, hospitals won over two-thirds of the elections.[6]

EXTENT OF UNIONIZATION IN THE THREE STATES

Given the differing legal frameworks for collective bargaining, the development of unionization should show important contrasts among the states as well as with what took place at the national level.

As American Hospital Association data for 1975 suggest, the extent of unionism varies greatly across the three states. On the one hand, Illinois had approximately the same number of hospitals with union contracts as the national average, 18.6 percent. Minnesota, where nearly half the hospitals had at least one labor agreement, greatly exceeded the national average. Wisconsin was at an intermediate point, with 26.1 percent.

Minnesota

Hospital collective bargaining was well established in Minnesota before the advent of federal control. By the mid-1940s, the Twin Cities of Minneapolis and St. Paul had become one of the only two centers of significant union strength in hospitals.[7] The other center was San Francisco. Actual or threatened strikes by hospital unions prompted the Minnesota legislature in 1947 to enact a separate law, the Charitable Hospitals Act, which covered all hospital workers except those employed in state hospitals.

The growth of unions over the years in Minnesota covered both professional and nonprofessional workers. Bargaining units which came into existence for the former group included RNs, LPNs, pharmacists, and radiologic technicians. In the latter category were service, maintenance, boiler room, and clerical employees. Thus, for example, in 1977 the Minnesota Nurses Association (MNA) claimed to represent 7,500 RNs working at 50 hospitals, and the Service Employees Union some 5,600 workers in 24 hospitals.

The success that health-care labor groups in Minnesota enjoyed over the years in organizing within their occupations and professions is readily apparent from Table 4.2. With the exception of therapists and medical technicians, the extent of unionization of professionals and technicians approached or exceeded 40 percent in 1976. In the other two states, the incidence of professional collective bargaining in hospitals was negligible. In addition, service and maintenance employees were well organized (40 percent or better). Only Wisconsin shows significant numbers of service workers unionized, and that at only half the rate of Minnesota.[†]

When the Taft-Hartley health-care amendments became law in 1974 there had already been many years of union activity in Minnesota

---

[†] It should be kept in mind that these are statewide totals. In cities such as Chicago and Minneapolis-St. Paul, the portion of workers unionized in each of the occupations and professions would be much larger.

hospitals. Thus, 46 percent of the nonprofit hospitals in the state
had one or more union contracts in contrast with 16 percent in Wisconsin, 9 percent in Illinois, and 13 percent for the United States
generally on that date. [8]

TABLE 4.2

Percentage of Occupations Unionized, 1976

	Wisconsin	Illinois	Minnesota	Total
Pharmacist	6.0	1.7	28.1	9.7
Therapist	2.9	1.9	0.0	1.7
RN	2.6	1.6	40.0	12.7
Nurses aide	23.0	11.1	37.5	21.8
LPN	15.4	1.6	41.0	16.5
Medical technician	2.6	1.7	2.6	2.2
Ward clerk	20.0	12.3	28.1	18.5
Maid	23.7	10.2	45.7	23.5
Kitchen helper	21.6	11.3	42.1	22.6
Stationary engineer	17.6	7.7	40.6	19.5
Switchboard operator	11.8	1.6	22.2	8.9
X-ray technician	8.1	5.5	29.6	14.1

Source: Mailed questionnaire of hospitals, 1976.

Examination of NLRB election data for the period August 1974
to July 1978 suggests that the number of organized hospitals, or
unionized employees in the private sector, did not change radically
in the post-health-care amendments period. Twenty-four elections
were held during those 48 months; unions were successful in 15 and,
as a result, 712 additional employees were brought under union contract. Whether recognized by election or voluntarily, approximately
52 percent of the 94 nonprofit hospitals of the state had union contracts.

In the public sector, the relevant statistics were 40 percent of
the federal and 32 percent of the state or local government hospitals
having some proportion of their hospital work forces organized.

The extent to which the larger hospitals comprise the backbone
of the unionized hospital labor force in Minnesota is revealed by the
following statistics: Among all hospitals, the average unionized hospital had 249 beds, while the average nonunion hospital had only 155.

Within the private, nonprofit sector, the differences were even greater; the average unionized hospital had 295 beds, while the average for a nonunion hospital was 160 beds.

Hospital collective bargaining was well dispersed geographically throughou the state in 1977. Only 25 of the 74 unionized hospitals are located in the Twin Cities area. This geographic distribution marks Minnesota as distinctly different from its two sister states, particularly Illinois.

Wisconsin

Hospital organizing activity began in earnest in Wisconsin in the mid-1950s, peaked in the period 1965-70, and tapered off thereafter. For example, from 1954 to 1963, unions were involved in 21 elections, winning 14 or 66.6 percent. [9] Election activity picked up during the following decade, with unions winning 31 of 75 representation elections (41 percent).

The main actor throughout the period after 1954 was Local 150 of the Service Employees International Union; this union was involved in eight elections in the early period and 45 in the later one. Other active unions were the International Brotherhood of Firemen and Oilers, the American Federation of State, County, and Municipal Employees (AFSCME), and the Wisconsin Nurses Association (WNA).

In the years since the Taft-Hartley amendments, 23 NLRB elections were held (to August 1978). Unions won 12, bringing an additional 848 workers under union contracts. It should be noted, however, that 386 bargaining unit members were brought under contract as a result of a single election.

By 1978, approximately 30 percent of the private, profit, and nonprofit hospitals in the state had union contracts. As in Minnesota, the unionized hospitals in Wisconsin tended (1) to be larger (50 percent of the unionized hospitals had 300 or more beds, whereas only 20 percent had fewer than 150); (2) to be in urbanized areas (only 15 percent of unionized hospitals were in communities with a population of 25,000 or less); and (3) not to be religiously affiliated.

In the public sector, two of the three federal hospitals were unionized, while at the state level, all hospitals run by the state of Wisconsin had one or more bargaining units. On the other hand, county and municipal hospitals were much less organized, with a rate of unionization approximating that of the private, nonprofit hospitals.

Illinois

As pointed out by Leo Osterhaus, "the history of the labor movement in the Chicago area is not as long nor as glorious as that of the San Francisco area, but it was turbulent during 1959-1960."[10] Apparently, only one labor contract had been negotiated at Chicago hospitals before that date, and that one by AFSCME.

In late 1959, under the direction of Victor Gotbaum, Local 1657 of AFSCME determined that Chicago hospitals were ready to be unionized and began with an organizing drive at Mt. Sinai hospital. In the midst of the campaign, two other unions entered the scene: Local 743 of the Teamsters and Local 73 of the Service Employees.[11] The unions' announced goal was a cooperative drive among themselves to organize virtually all hospitals in the Chicago metropolitan area.

For two months AFSCME sought recognition from Mt. Sinai and the Chicago Home for the Incurables and then struck the hospitals in August 1959. Five months later the strike ended unsuccessfully for the union.

Simultaneously with the activity of AFSCME, Teamsters Local 743 began its own drive, seeking recognition from a number of other hospitals. Although this union threatened further strikes, none took place and the hospitals remained nonunion.

Despite the unions' professed intention of cooperating in their organizing drives, they did not. AFSCME's picket lines were not honored by other unions, including the Teamsters, and Local 73 "was accused of trying behind the scenes to prevent some hospitals from recognizing [either] Teamsters, Local 743 or AFSCME, Local 1657."[12]

Many factors combined to block the unionizing drives of 1959 to 1960, including the lack of legal protection for organizing and bargaining and a loose labor market that provided an ample supply of replacements for strikers. The major deterrent apparently was the organizational rivalry among the three unions. When efforts to unionize Chicago hospitals were resumed in the mid-1960s, this lesson was not lost.

In the summer of 1966, the heads of Teamsters Local 743 and Service Employees Local 73 met to plan a renewed hospital-organizing campaign. Out of this meeting was born Health Employees Labor Program, a joint organization supported by both unions. HELP's proclaimed focus was private sector health-care institutions, leaving the public sector to AFSCME or other public employee unions.[13] Also, because the leaders were persuaded that professionals could be unionized only after the nonprofessionals were, they decided to limit HELP's jurisdiction to the nonprofessional employees. Most of the nonprofessional hospital workers were minority group members whose incomes were at the poverty level, and in an era of great social upheaval, the union campaigns had civil rights implications. In May 1967, HELP won an important election at one of the largest private hospitals in Chicago, Presbyterian-St. Lukes.[14]

The "Pres-St. Lukes" success was a springboard into many other Chicago hospitals to the extent that by 1971 HELP held contracts in 18 hospitals. Through 1975, five additional hospitals were unionized, bringing under union contract more than 7,000 members in 23 Chicago area hospitals.[15] The foundation was now constructed on which not only professionals but also hospital employees in both the public and private sectors beyond Chicago could be unionized. However, this expectation was not realized in the immediate future for reasons to be examined below.

Approximately 15 percent of the state's 245 short-term community hospitals had union contracts in 1977, but this figure obscures several very important characteristics of hospital labor relations in Illinois. First, there was a very heavy concentration of union hospitals in Chicago, the proportion exceeding 75 percent. Second, even the suburbs of Chicago remained virtually impervious to union-organizing drives; only 7 percent of them employed unionized workers. Although it is arguable, some observers believe that HELP's identification with the civil rights movement and its high proportion of minority members were drawbacks in mounting effective organizing drives in Chicago's predominantly white suburbs.

Many of the trends noted earlier were also evident in Illinois. Thus, for example, only 12 percent of the state's religiously affiliated hospitals had contracts, although this proportion was 39 percent in Chicago. The larger hospitals, as measured by number of beds, were more apt to be unionized. The average union hospital in metropolitan Chicago had 462 beds, and its nonunion counterpart only 261.

Public sector hospitals shared many of the characteristics identified previously with federal, state, or local institutions in Wisconsin and Minnesota. Federal hospitals were well organized in Illinois; only one of seven had no labor agreement. Although six of the eight public hospitals (75 percent) in the Chicago metropolitan area were unionized, only 7 percent of state, county, or municipal hospitals in the remainder of Illinois had collective contracts.

In the private sector, at least, it is clear that a plateau of union growth in Illinois hospitals was reached in the early 1970s, perhaps even before the Taft-Hartley amendments took effect. HELP, for example, was successful in only one out of six organizing efforts between January 1972 and August 1974. In the aftermath of the assumption of federal jurisdiction, hospital union membership in Illinois did not expand appreciably. Although 47 elections took place, unions were successful in only 13 during the period for which data are available (August 1974 to July 1978). Consequently, 1,163 workers came under labor contracts, more than half of these as a result of just two elections.[16]

As indicated in Table 4.2, union organization is concentrated almost totally among nonprofessional hospital employees in Illinois. By 1976, the Illinois Nurses Association (INA) had been successful in organizing only one private hospital. It held two contracts in public hospitals, and had a 1,050-member unit in the Illinois Department of Mental Health. The Licensed Practical Nurses Association also was generally restricted to the public sector, although "statements of understanding" did exist with several of the larger private hospitals.

Unions holding scattered bargaining units, particularly among craft workers, included the operating engineers, carpenters, plumbers, electrical workers (International Brotherhood of Electrical Workers), firemen and oilers, and machinists (International Association of Machinists). These craft units frequently were relatively informal in nature and often were covered only by the "statements of understanding."

CONCLUDING THOUGHTS ON UNIONISM IN THE THREE STATES

In retrospect, it is clear that the 1974 Taft-Hartley amendments did not have a marked effect on the level of unionization across the three states. The growth in the number of hospital bargaining units tapered off in the early 1970s, and the changes in the federal law did not stimulate a new surge.

Moreover, in projecting changes in hospital unionization, one is tempted to predict that, at least in the near future, the level will not increase dramatically. On the one hand, with the larger city hospitals in the three states now organized, the smaller, rural, and church-affiliated institutions pose a formidable challenge. Smaller hospitals often have much higher proportions of part-time and voluntary workers who may see no advantage in joining unions or supporting collective bargaining. The social climate in small towns or rural areas also often attaches negative values to unionism, particularly if it appears to emanate from other geographical areas and/or ethnic groups.

The increasing sophistication of hospital managements and their use of outside consultants to counter union-organizing drives are other barriers to unionization. The intricacies of the legal framework and lengthy appeal procedures to the NLRB make it possible to contest representation issues over many months, perhaps "chilling" the desire of employees to engage in collective action.

On the other hand, the unions themselves appear to be in a passive state in the late 1970s. Certain unions, particularly among nonprofessional employees, seem to have occupied early the "commanding heights" and once having done so, are unable or unwilling to move out aggressively.

For other unions, success in the Midwest has been much more difficult to achieve than on their home grounds. Thus, District 1199 of New York has not been able to extend a small foothold in a few nursing homes into a successful drive on hospitals. The same is true of the Retail Clerks and the Laborers. The near monopoly position acquired by SEIU and HELP among nonprofessional employees is a major obstacle.

The level of unionization of the professional employees is even less likely to change. The associations still confront severe internal crises in which supervisors and hospital administrators often continue to exercise significant influence over association policy. Even when collective bargaining is accepted association policy, individual members tend to reject such a role as "nonprofessional." The values of "Nightingaleism" still hold sway. For the numerically smaller professional occupations such as pharmacist and therapist, the NLRB has virtually foreclosed collective bargaining except through a coalition. Diverse interests and professional jealousies stand in the way of collective coordinated action for the time being.

Moreover, in the case of registered nurses, recent decisions by the federal courts have raised serious questions concerning the ability of either the national or state nurses associations to continue representing RNs for bargaining purposes under the National Labor Relations Act. In the landmark case Anne Arundel Hospital, the Fourth Circuit Court of Appeals struck down a long-standing policy of the NLRB by which state associations could be certified as bargaining representatives provided the actual negotiations were delegated to a local hospital chapter.[17] The rationale for the NLRB's action had been the fact that nursing educators and administrators occupied a predominant role in policy-making positions at the state and national level of the nursing associations. The federal court concluded it was "illogical and illegal" to certify a bargaining agent on the condition it not bargain.

While the national association has struggled with the formulation of policy to meet the objections of Anne Arundel, the state associations have had to confront the immediate practical consequences of the court's decision. In the case of Wisconsin, for example, hospital employers have threatened lengthy litigation in representation elections in which the Wisconsin Nurses Association appeared on the ballot.[18] In addition, the possibility has increased that as existing contracts held by the WNA expire administrators will refuse to engage in negotiations to renew the agreements.

In order to avoid such disputes, the Wisconsin Nurses Association, acting through its House of Delegates, voted in December 1978 to cease its collective bargaining activities for registered nurses in the state.[19] The WNA's decision immediately spawned a new group, United Professionals for Quality Health Care (UP), which sought to replace WNA in the latter's 19 bargaining units. The financial backing for United Professionals was supplied by the Wisconsin Education Association Council, a National Education Association affiliate, and the chief organizer for UP had formerly been a staff member of WNA.

The events taking place in Wisconsin were foreshadowed in Connecticut, New Jersey, Michigan, and California where dissident RNs have broken away to form independent organizations dedicated almost exclusively to collective bargaining activities. Illustrative of these trends are the United Nurses Association of California and the Connecticut Health Care Association.

Nationally, the picture is further clouded by the efforts of such unions as the Service Employees International, District 1199, AFSCME, and most recently the American Federation of Teachers to gain bargaining rights among registered nurses.[20] At the end of 1978 these particular labor organizations had made no visible moves to replace the state nursing associations as bargaining representatives in any of the three states studied here.

Moreover, unlike their sister association in Wisconsin, the nursing associations of Illinois and Minnesota have expressed their intention of continuing their present collective bargaining policies. Only if legal action ultimately forces them to do so will the MNA and INA withdraw from the health-care labor-management arena. In the meantime, there is also the hope that Anne Arundel will be reversed in other cases still pending in the federal courts.

In summary then, from the unions' standpoint it is a bleak picture across the three states. From August 1974 through July 1978, unions won just 40 of 94 elections, or 42.5 percent. This rate is significantly lower than the national industry average, as well as that for all hospital elections in the United States. For all their efforts, the combined total number of workers organized in private, nonprofit hospitals in Illinois, Wisconsin, and Minnesota since the amendments took effect in 1974 was 2,682. Some 9,931 employees were involved in elections that unions lost. Union concern with federal labor policy that opposes fragmentation of bargaining units seems to be borne out if one examines the outcome of elections by size of bargaining unit. The average bargaining unit in the elections lost numbered 184 employees; in elections won, it numbered 67.

NOTES

1. As calculated from statistics presented in Hervey Juris et al., "Nationwide Survey Shows Growth in Union Contracts," Hospitals, JAHA 51 (March 16, 1977): 125, table 1.

2. See Paul D. Frenzen, "Survey Updates Unionization Activities," Hospitals, JAHA 52 (August 1, 1978): 94.

3. Office of Wages and Industrial Relations, Bureau of Labor Statistics, personal communication to the authors, December 13, 1978.

4. Joseph Rosmann, "One Year Under Taft-Hartley," Hospitals, JAHA 49 (December 16, 1975): 64.

5. Calculated from NLRB, Monthly Report, August 1974–December 1977.

6. See Rosmann, "One Year Under Taft-Hartley," p. 66.

7. Ronald L. Miller, "Collective Bargaining in Non-Profit Hospitals" (Ph.D. diss., University of Pennsylvania, 1969), pp. 17–18.

8. Office of Technical Services (Unpublished report, FMCS, August 7, 1974), table 1. There are no for profit hospitals in Minnesota.

9. Archives of the Wisconsin Employment Relations Commission.

10. Leo B. Osterhaus, "Labor Unions in the Hospital and Their Effect on Management" (Ph.D. diss., University of Texas at Austin, 1966), p. 146.

11. Ibid.

12. Ibid., p. 152.

13. Norman Metzger and Dennis D. Pointer, Labor Management Relations in the Health Services Industry: Theory and Practice (Washington, D.C.: Science and Health, 1972), pp. 32–34.

14. See Analysis of Collective Bargaining Agreements in Chicago Area Hospitals, 1975–76 (Chicago: Chicago Hospital Council, 1975), p. 3.

15. Ibid., p. 2.

16. National Labor Relations Board, Monthly Election Reports, August 1974–July 1978.

17. NLRB v. Anne Arundel Emergency Hospital Association d/b/a Anne Arundel General Hospital, CA 4, No. 76-1166, August 31, 1977.

18. An interview with representatives of the Wisconsin Nurses Association revealed that in one such case involving Bellin Memorial Hospital of Green Bay, Wisconsin, the WNA was forced to withdraw from a representation election as a consequence of the employer's objections. The hospital contended the fact that the

incoming president of the WNA also occupied a management role in Bellin Hospital constituted a conflict of interest and negated the WNA's claim to be a legitimate labor organization.

19. John Junkerman, "Area Nurses Forge New Union," The Madison Press Connection, December 11, 1978, pp. 2-3.

20. See, for example, "Teacher Union Seeks to Organize Workers in Health Professions," New York Times, November 30, 1978, p. A15.

5

HOSPITAL BARGAINING
RELATIONSHIPS: STRUCTURE,
PROCESS, AND ISSUES

Over the years, collective bargaining has been variously defined as a system for marketing labor, an exercise in industrial democracy, or a procedure for joint decision making of the rules and policies that bind employees and employers together.[1] Whatever the concept, each seems to contain the premise that the relationships of labor and management will be structured in a relatively formal fashion, usually with identifiable and regularized roles, status hierarchies, authority relationships, and rules in the tradition of Max Weber. In addition, as an outgrowth of the structuring of the relationships, there will also be a process by which decisions of a procedural and substantive nature can be made and implemented.

In the early stages of the union-employer relationship, structural and procedural questions may predominate. Thus, issues needing resolution at that point may deal with such matters as who is entitled to act as representative for employees or management, on what basis may they speak, and for which subjects. Where the parties have been in disagreement on the means of deciding such questions, public bodies often have intervened to assist—or compel—mutual agreement. The structure of the labor-management relationships thus reflects the needs and goals of the parties and is a means to an end.

To the degree that a collective bargaining relationship affects other systems or relationships in the broader society, external pressures may become important. For example, a wage increase in a single establishment may go unnoticed, while the same wage increase across an entire industry or region may have immediate political and social implications. Work stoppages or lockouts provide even stronger illustrations of these tendencies.

BARGAINING RELATIONSHIPS IN
THE HOSPITAL INDUSTRY

More so than many other industries, health care in general and hospitals in particular present a complex picture of bureaucratic and administrative systems. "Management" is a composite of administrators, medical staff, and trustees, each exercising varying amounts of decision-making authority. Moreover, in recent years, the administrative process has become subject to numerous outside bodies including accreditation and licensing agencies, rate review commissions, and health-planning organizations, not to mention those directly concerned with employee matters such as the Equal Employment Opportunities Commission (EEOC), the NLRB, and the legions of ERISA, OSHA, FLSA, and so forth.[†]

Moreover, the hospital industry is one in which more than 90 percent of the operating revenues are derived from public and private insurance programs. Consequently, competitive market forces do not affect the sale of health services by the average public or private, nonprofit hospital.[2]

In the context of the hospital, therefore, it is not accurate to speak of collective bargaining as joint or bilateral decision making. Rather, it is multilateral or multiparty.[3] In this respect, hospital bargaining bears only a superficial resemblance to traditional private sector industrial relations.

HOSPITAL BARGAINING STRUCTURES

The discussion of hospital collective bargaining structures presented here will follow from the definition provided by Arnold Weber, who argues:

> It is apparent that collective bargaining structure cannot be identified with any simple notion of bargaining unit. Instead, a given collective bargaining structure is composed of a _multiplicity_ of units tied together in a complicated network of relationships by social, legal, and administrative factors.[4]

[†] These are the Employment Retirement Income Security Act, the Occupational Safety and Health Act, and the Fair Labor Standards Act.

Four types of bargaining units that were identified are (1) informal work groups, (2) election districts, (3) negotiation units, and (4) the units of direct impact. In the remaining pages of this section, Weber's framework, modified slightly, will be used to examine the hospital bargaining relationships in the three states.

Informal Bargaining Units

Bargaining relationships may come into existence lacking formal legalization, but nevertheless with important practical significance. Groups may be organized around age, ethnic or racial factors, sex, shift assignments, or occupation. In addition, they may provide the foundation for the development of other components of the bargaining structure, including election districts and negotiating units.

Across the three states, numerous illustrations of informal bargaining units came to light during the course of the study. In Chicago, the role of blacks as the cohesive force in eventually building a successful labor movement (HELP) has already been noted. Generally, the high proportion of females in a given occupation, such as nursing, may also be an important tie binding a group together for bargaining.

Often the occupation itself is a major factor around which individuals coalesce for either informal or formal collective action. Notable here are such groups as residents and interns (housestaff) working through committees in some hospitals, and LPNs and craft workers, who at times may be covered by little more than memorandums or "statements of understanding." A specific illustration in Minnesota is that of the nurse anesthetist, an occupation limited to registered nurses with two years of specialized training and subject to certification by the American Association of Nurse Anesthetists. They were not part of the RN bargaining unit administered by the Minnesota Nurses Association.

Nurse Anesthetists in the Twin Cities area desired more voice in the determination of their wages, and the bargaining representative for the majority of Twin City hospitals, Health Manpower Management Incorporated (HMMI), after discussing the issue, agreed to study the situation. The result was not a formal contract, but mutual agreement of HMMI and the nurse anesthetists on a base rate and a new method of payment.

Several factors may contribute to informal bargaining within hospital election districts and negotiating units in the future. First, the policy of the NLRB to permit only broad representation units composed of service and maintenance workers, technicians, and all nonnursing professionals is lumping together many employees with only a minimal "community of interest." Carpenters, electricians, stationary engineers, X-ray technicians, LPNs, and pharmacists, for example, have their own unions or associations and are accustomed to separate treatment.

Second, economic, administrative, and technological pressures are combined to impel mergers of hospitals, to stimulate expanded geographical planning of the delivery of health-care services, and to standardize evaluation and treatment by a host of public and semipublic regulatory bodies. Decision-making authority is gradually moving upward and away from the individual local hospital.

Finally, the bargaining structure of the parties, particularly on labor's side, is already quite centralized and geographically broad, with a single local union often responsible for the negotiation and administration of collective bargaining agreements in many different hospitals.

The consequence of these diverse factors is to make the locus of collective bargaining decision-making power increasingly remote from the individual worker in a hospital. Further, as more diverse groups and occupations become represented under a single contract, the terms of agreement may, of necessity, become quite general. As a result, a good deal of informal bargaining may eventually result in trying to "fit" the contract to the point of application. "Side" agreements or informal understandings may, in fact, become the reality of the everyday hospital work situation, apart from and, perhaps, in contradiction to the rules or stipulations officially provided in a master contract.

Election Districts

Often labeled as the "appropriate bargaining unit," the election district is created either by the NLRB or the relevant state labor board, depending upon the specific political jurisdiction in question. In Illinois the parties themselves largely negotiated their own election units before 1974. In Wisconsin and Minnesota, the Wisconsin Employment Relations Commission and the Bureau of Mediation Services, respectively, usually performed this function.

Congress's admonition to the NLRB at the time of the passage of health-care amendments to Taft-Hartley revealed widespread concern over the scope of administratively determined election units. It was felt that the state boards often had carved out units whose narrow boundaries provided for intransigent problems of jurisdictional conflict over occupational boundaries, barriers to efficient and flexible use of manpower, and "unbalanced" wage structures. Also cited were such potential problems as interunion rivalry in bargaining, work interruptions from limited picketing, and work stoppages being generalized from a small group to an entire hospital complex.

In New York State, for example, despite the fact that the State Labor Relations Board initially attempted to limit the number to five, eventually 12 or more units became certified in some hospitals. Minnesota was another example of unit fragmentation, with election districts certified by the state Bureau of Mediation Services for pharmacists, radiologic technologists, LPNs, RNs, service workers, stationary engineers, maintenance employees, and clerical workers, among others. As one observer aptly describes it, such situations are ripe for occupational tribalism in hospital work forces.[5]

In Wisconsin and Illinois, little organizing activity occurred among registered nurses and other professional workers before 1974. Some initiative existed among craft workers, but it was sporadic and, at times, limited to informal bargaining. Thus, although the WERC, for its part, may have been prepared to follow the unit policy of its sister board in Minnesota, few occasions to do so arose.

In view of the above, it is not surprising that an examination of the amount of unit proliferation discloses great variation between Minnesota and the other two states. As Table 5.1 reveals, approximately 60 percent of Minnesota hospitals have two or more contracts. Wisconsin and Illinois, on the other hand, are characterized by one-unit hospitals.

Another way to measure unit proliferation is to place a hospital's work force into 12 categories[†] and then examine how many of these categories are covered by a particular hospital labor agreement. Drawing upon data supplied by the American Hospital Association, we find that 66 percent of Wisconsin hospital contracts cover two or more of the 12 categories; in Illinois the figure is 50 percent, and in Minnesota only 25 percent.

If there is occupational tribalism in hospitals, it is obviously less prevalent in Wisconsin and Illinois than in Minnesota. Moreover, unless the NLRB unit determination policy changes radically,

---

[†]The categories are service; maintenance; technical employees; plant clerical; office clerical; housestaff; physician, professional registered nurse; licensed practical nurse; security guard; and supervisor.

TABLE 5.1

Distribution of Hospitals with One or More Bargaining Units, 1976

Number of Units Per Hospital	Wisconsin		Illinois		Minnesota	
	Number of Hospitals	Percent of Total	Number of Hospitals	Percent of Total	Number of Hospitals	Percent of Total
1	25	75.7	20	80.0	15	33.3
2	6	18.1	3	12.0	6.	13.3
3	2	6.2	1	4.0	7	15.6
4	0	0	1	4.0	1	2.2
5	0	0	0	0	6	13.3
6	0	0	0	0	9	20.0
7	0	0	0	0	1	2.2
Total	33	100.0	25	100.0	45	100.0

Note: Although a diligent search was undertaken of all available sources, it is likely that the count of bargaining units presented in the table understates slightly the total number of such units as well as the number per hospital.

Source: Mailed questionnaire of hospitals, 1976.

unit proliferation is not likely to rise in future years. How much impact the existing unit configuration has on bargaining will be discussed later.

Negotiation Units

The continuing concern over election unit proliferation overlooks the fact that the bargaining or negotiating unit frequently is not synonymous with that established by certification or election. Although few would accept the extreme position taken by John Dunlop that, except for a few situations, the bargaining unit established by the NLRB has little relevance to bargaining,[6] it is true that quite often bargaining may go on within the election unit ("fractional bargaining," in Neil Chamberlain's phrase), or beyond the original unit in a multiemployer or multiunion negotiating structure.

Formal multiemployer negotiating units are a significant characteristic of hospital bargaining in Minnesota, although not in the other two states. Thus, for example, the Minnesota Nurses Association has RNs covered by labor agreements at more than 50 hospitals. One contract, however, encompasses 23 hospitals alone. For SEIU Local 113, the situation is quite similar, with 5,000 of its total 5,500 members covered under one 22-hospital negotiating unit. In fact, almost regardless of the craft, skill level, or profession involved, in Minnesota it is highly probable that employees will be represented by a large multihospital unit. This is especially true if the hospital is located in Minneapolis-St. Paul.

Illinois and Wisconsin, on the other hand, do not have any private sector, multihospital negotiating units. Such groups as the Chicago Hospital Association and the Greater Milwaukee Hospital Association supply labor relations services but do not have authority to bargain for their member hospitals.

The absence of multiemployer bargaining in Illinois and Wisconsin appears to reflect practices in the United States generally, except for the Bay Area of San Francisco, New York City, and Seattle.[7] In fact, about 85 percent of unionized hospitals in the tristate area had single-hospital negotiating units.[8]

Why should multihospital bargaining exist in some areas and not others? A possible explanation is that in the pre-1974 period hospitals in urban areas seem to have been vulnerable to "whipsawing" by unions, a bargaining tactic of singling out the weakest employer in a competitive industry and attempting to play one enterprise off against the others, pyramiding the terms reached in each agreement. Hence, multiemployer or association bargaining was a strategy of solidarity and is considered by some management bargainers as the "countersaw" to the "whipsaw."[9]

Hospitals in group bargaining situations usually agree to exchange relevant information affecting wages, hours, and working conditions, engage in a uniform approach to union and nonunion employees alike, develop a single position in recognition and negotiating matters, select one spokesperson for the group, adopt a joint strategy, coordinate publicity, and give each other lawful aid or assistance.[10] Hospitals may go so far as to pool resources and share the costs of labor relations specialists.

The benefits thus are many for those hospitals that participate in a full "countersaw." The costs are also high, and for this reason hospitals may stop short of becoming a part of an association negotiating unit. For example, the individual hospital must accept whatever bargaining outcome is attained by the association. For hospitals in a marginal economic position, contractual wage settlements may be too high or constraints on the use of personnel too stringent. In contrast, the largest hospital may not want to be tied to the "lowest common denominator" of the industry and, in fact, may feel it can get a better deal by bargaining independently. In either case, group bargaining represents a loss of management discretion and autonomy that can outweigh the benefits of countersawing.

Unlike the Twin City hospitals represented by HMMI, those of Chicago and Milwaukee have chosen the independent road of negotiating. They join together in their respective associations for all the other activities cited above, while continuing to refrain from taking the final step.

When and if the final step to full association bargaining will occur is a matter for speculation. On the one hand, the pressures to consolidate election districts and negotiating units are becoming increasingly strong. On the other, the present inability of the hospital unions in the three states to mount effective organizing and bargaining activities reduces the necessity of giving up individual control in exchange for group protection. Whipsawing is, as yet, not a sufficient threat to justify a countersaw strategy.

The Units of Direct Impact

In the same way that the boundaries of the negotiating unit may extend considerably beyond the original election district, so too the effects of the negotiation activities may be transmitted to other parties, some unionized and some not. Arthur Ross many years ago coined the phrase "orbits of coercive comparison" to describe the dynamics of this phenomenon.[11]

One major orbit of coercive comparison is the hospital association, which provides a mechanism by which wage and other information can be exchanged and, in certain instances, wage settlements imposed even on nonunion hospital members. A second orbit is the union, which, in the hospital industry, often has a wide geographic base in addition to a particular class of workers. This point will be examined more fully in a later section of the chapter. Suffice it to say, however, that the geographic basis by which the hospital industry union is organized enables it to make interhospital wage comparisons easily and to develop a standardized bargaining strategy for industrywide or areawide rates, prevailing wages, union scales, and so forth. In addition, such unions as the Service Employees and the Operating Engineers, among others, generally represent workers of approximately the same skill level in non-health-care enterprises and industries. Thus, for example, the standard wage for stationary engineers expected by the IUOE at a hospital may be that which is paid to similar employees organized by the union in the local area's large office buildings.

As might be expected, pattern bargaining is the norm within the industry. Among professionals, a contract settlement among nurses may induce other professional groups to follow suit formally or for the hospital administration to make adjustments to keep salary structures in balance. In addition, larger hospitals may generate "key" bargains with its contract settlements that then carry over to the often smaller, satellite hospitals.

The late arrival and relatively low incidence of hospital unionism tend to reinforce the system of pattern bargaining between as well as within hospitals. In the face of the possibility or threat of unionization, nonunion hospitals may modify their wages and working conditions as these change with new contracts in the unionized sector of the industry. In this way, the hospital may hope to undermine a union's campaign to persuade the hospital's employees that there are benefits from supporting the union. The impact of collective bargaining on compensation in hospitals and the role of the so-called threat effect will be examined in Chapter 7.

THE PARTIES' BARGAINING STRUCTURE

Management

Although in the majority of cases hospital management conducted its own bargaining, several exceptions to this pattern should be noted. First, hospital councils play what appears to be an increasingly important role, particularly in the larger urban areas. In all but the Twin Cities, individual hospitals continue to retain their bargaining autonomy and final decision-making discretion while otherwise sharing information and coordinating strategy.

Over the long run, however, many signs point to the multi-hospital replacing the single hospital as a negotiating unit. Therefore, it is useful to examine at this point one such multimanagement bargaining arrangement, Health Manpower Management. The roots of HMMI go back to the late 1930s and the existence of the Hospital Council of Minneapolis. The council and its counterpart in St. Paul provided a meeting place for administrators and other hospital managers who were facing a series of organizing drives among the city's nonprofessional hospital employees by the SEIU Local 113. One of these administrators had come from the hotel industry where multiemployer bargaining was customary.

It was clear to the hospital administrators, particularly from 1953 on, that if they were to avoid being whipsawed, they had to coordinate their individual hospital activities. Such coordination, much the same as is currently practiced by the Chicago Hospital Council (CHC) and the Greater Milwaukee Hospital Council, was carried out until 1972 under the aegis of what had by then become the Twin Cities Hospital Council.

Born out of the old Twin Cities council in 1972, HMMI had the power to negotiate for, but not to bind, member institutions. Each hospital retained its right to accept or reject the final master agreement. It is asserted that a schism within the ranks of the LPN association in Minnesota, which raised the specter of a civil war between the two LPN factions, persuaded previously reluctant administrators to cede ultimate authority in negotiating to HMMI. Under current membership rules, if a majority of hospitals belonging to HMMI ratifies a contract, a member hospital must accept the contract or withdraw from the group.

Loss of membership could be a major blow to an individual hospital. HMMI undertakes wage surveys and studies of specialized topics such as turnover but, most importantly, directly negotiates collective agreements either on a multimanagement basis or for individual hospitals. The latter system prevails for "corresponding" members who receive consulting or negotiating services for a flat fee.

Bargaining teams usually consist of the two staff professionals from Health Manpower Management, two hospital administrators, several personnel administrators, a few nursing supervisors, and, as spokesperson and chief negotiator, an attorney from a law firm closely associated with HMMI. The exact composition of the bargaining team varies with the contract being negotiated. Noncompliance with negotiated contract terms by member institutions appears to have been minimal and, thus, provides a measure of the success achieved by HMMI.

From the hospitals' standpoint, other measures of success are an almost total lack of strikes since the early 1950s and a salary and benefits level that has risen very slowly in recent years in contrast to comparable unionized hospitals in other parts of the country. In the late 1940s and early 1950s, the rates for registered nurses and nonprofessionals were higher than for similar hospital employees elsewhere. Salaries, however, have risen more rapidly since that time in such cities as San Francisco, and now the Twin Cities' rates lag considerably behind.

A second major pattern of bargaining structure on the hospital side is the prevalence of attorneys in key negotiating roles. A lawyer is the chief spokesperson for the HMMI negotiating team. In both the hospital councils and individual hospitals, lawyers appear to shape the labor relations policies. More often than not, they are not hospital employees but consultants on retainer from firms specializing in providing legal services to employers with labor problems. Services may range from advice during election campaigns, representation before the NLRB and the courts, preparation of briefs for arbitration hearings, and direct participation in the bargaining itself.

The prevalence of attorneys is not unexpected, given the late and incomplete unionization of the hospital industry. At the present time, a majority of hospital administrators and trustees believe that hospitals function most efficiently without interference from unions. In addition, many hospital administrators are inexperienced in labor relations in general, and they find themselves in a situation where legal regulation of all aspects of the industry is pervasive and complex.

Further, the "cost-pass-through" system by which the industry has been financed in recent years has provided funds not only to keep wages and benefits up in the face of threats to unionized hospitals but also has created a mechanism for meeting the expenses incurred in purchasing labor relations services and advice. With cost constraints and rate reviews now becoming generalized, the ease with which this aspect of a hospital's operating cost can be "passed on" may be significantly reduced.

Finally, one suspects that as hospital managements acquire training and expertise, they may be less inclined to delegate labor relations activity and policies to outside experts. In this respect, the continuing need for legal services may be supplied by attorneys employed directly by the hospital or, more likely, by the council to which the hospital belongs.

Union

Just as with management, the labor organization structure for bargaining exhibits strong centralizing characteristics. Hospital employees tend to be incorporated in local unions whose jurisdictions are not only occupational in nature but also geographically extensive in scope. For example, SEIU Locals 113 and 150 in Minnesota and Wisconsin, respectively, cover nearly the whole state. Local 113, with a staff of less than four full-time persons, services 45 to 50 hospitals in which it has members under contract; 5,000 members in 22 hospitals are covered by one contract. Although there is no large multihospital unit in Wisconsin, Local 150's situation is quite similar.

The structure of the associations of professional employees is also geographically extensive in all three states. The Minnesota Nurses Association holds bargaining rights over 6,000 RNs in some 50 to 55 hospitals. Like its nonprofessional union counterpart, Local 113, half these members are in a single negotiating unit of 22 hospitals.

There are both strong similarities and important differences in union organization in Chicago. (Little will be said about the remainder of Illinois since its rate of hospital unionization is so low.) The major health-care labor organization in Illinois's largest city is the joint creation of Teamsters Local 743 and Service Employees 73, the Health Employees Labor Program.

HELP constitutes an independent labor organization, unaffiliated and with its own constitution, bylaws, and officers. It is controlled totally, however, by the founding unions, which supply its executive board members and its administrative officers. For example, it is customary to alternate the president and secretary-treasurer positions between Locals 743 and 73.[12] In addition, as hospitals are unionized, the new union members are divided equally between the two locals. If these new members are to influence the bargaining policy of HELP, they must do so through the parent Locals 743 or 73.

HELP had a meteoric rise, achieving recognition from 23 hospitals between 1966 and 1972. However, since 1972 it has been for the most part unsuccessful, both in its attempts to unionize within Chicago and in the suburbs and also in its efforts to organize professional and clerical workers beyond its normally nonprofessional base.

Observers attribute its lack of success to several factors. HELP's identification as a largely nonprofessional, ethnically oriented union has hindered its acceptance by professional workers and those outside Chicago. The determination of the Chicago Hospital Council and related hospitals to prevent unionization has been a second factor. Third, other unions, even locals within the parent Teamsters and Service Employees, have also mounted organizing drives, thus undercutting HELP's efforts. Finally, with the right to strike for recognition effectively removed by the federal labor law, HELP has lost a major element of its bargaining power.

The weakness of its position is perhaps best illustrated by the willingness of CHC hospitals to continue to bargain on a separate and independent basis. The whipsaw which was so strong a factor in impelling hospitals in the Twin Cities, San Francisco, and elsewhere is missing from the Chicago hospital scene.

ROLE OF THIRD PARTIES IN BARGAINING

Much has already been made of the fact that hospital bargaining is a multiparty process. Increasingly, the so-called third-party payer has acquired a role in bargaining, influencing, or even controlling contract settlements.[13] Although third parties have become important to the negotiations in the Northeast, they have not yet achieved a similar position in any of the three states investigated here. Neither the private insurance organizations nor the government agencies has played a significant role in bargaining.

The reasons for the absence of third parties are not clear but undoubtedly reflect the more favorable financial situation of both the public sector and the hospital industry in the upper Midwest. Bargaining settlements have been mostly conservative, not likely to constitute unmanageable pressures on health-care costs.

Forces external to the hospital labor-management relationship, however, may interject third parties, particularly as public authorities bring under review all aspects of hospital operation, whether it be capital acquisition, building programs, services provided, or rates charged. The logic of the situation would not seem to provide control for one set of factors affecting hospital costs while at the same time overlooking those derived from labor.

INSTITUTIONAL FACTORS AFFECTING
BARGAINING STRUCTURE

After the labor-management relationship has been created, the parties may pursue certain goals in their bargaining to strengthen their relative positions. Typically, these are clauses dealing with management rights and union security. Contractual attainment of these goals may reinforce the company or the union as an institution, insuring its survival and enabling it to concentrate its efforts on other bargaining ends.

Management Rights

Administrators themselves are not of one mind regarding the value of including a management rights clause in a contract. Some fear that including such a clause in a bargaining agreement itself casts doubts about the "rights" of management; others insist that no contract is complete without such a clause. All recognize that problems may arise from the inadvertent omission of a function or activity from a list of management rights, thus raising a barrier to an employer's unhampered exercise of that function.

Hospital managers do not differ from those of other industries in their disagreement over the value of a management rights clause. In the tristate area, approximately 60 percent of the hospital contracts contain such a clause.[14]

Union Security

Although they are not precise parallels, a contractual requirement that stipulates union membership as a condition of employment is often considered to be labor's counterpart of the management rights clause. Union security clauses appear in many forms including (1) union shop, which provides a grace period often corresponding to time spent as a probationary employee before a worker must join the union as a condition of employment; (2) modified union shop, in which current employees may exercise an option to stay out of the union, but those newly hired must join; (3) agency shop, which allows voluntary membership but requires payment of fees equivalent to the union's dues; and (4) those where maintenance of membership is not compulsory, but continued membership is expected for at least the duration of the contract. As Hervey Juris points out, "The inclusion of strong union security provisions in a contract is a basic measure of union power."[15] Dues collection is facilitated and discipline over members may be more effectively enforced.

When compared on the criterion of strength of the union security provision, as in Table 5.2, unions in Illinois, Minnesota, and Wisconsin have not achieved as much bargaining power as hospital unions elsewhere in the country and possess much less than unions in other industries. [†]

If, from the research of Hervey Juris and his associates, it were possible to disaggregate the contract analysis by control of hospital and by occupation, it is likely that the combined data for

---

[†] It should be noted that none of the three states in question has exercised its option under Section 14B of the Labor Management Relations Act to prohibit union security.

the three states would show important differences. First, union security would be more prevalent in private sector than public sector hospitals.[16] If it occurred in the public sector, it would be in the form of the agency shop rather than the union shop, which is most frequently found in private hospitals.

TABLE 5.2

Distribution of Union Security Agreements in the
Tristate Area and the United States, 1976
(in percentage of contracts)

Contract Provision	Hospitals in Combined Three States (N = 126 contracts)	All U.S. (N = 504 contracts)	Nonhospital Industries
Union shop	28.0	31.0	63.0
Modified union shop	8.0	9.0	11.0
Agency shop	3.0	13.0	4.0
Maintenance of membership	20.0	13.0	4.0
No union security	40.0	34.0	18.0

Sources: Combined three states: personal communication to the authors from the Training and Employee Relations Department, American Hospital Association. All U.S. hospitals and other industries: Bureau of National Affairs, Daily Labor Report, no. 116 (June 15, 1976), p. A3.

Second, union security clauses are more apt to be missing from the contracts of professional employees than from those of nonprofessionals. For the latter group, the union shop seems to be more easily attainable; for other groups, the lesser forms of security may be equally represented. Finally, union security, generally in its strongest forms, seems to be associated more often with the larger nonprofit, non-church-associated, urban hospitals than with contracts in institutions lacking these characteristics.

Dues Checkoff

Automatic deduction of union dues and fees is a dimension of
union security that strengthens a union's bargaining position significantly. With a continuing flow of funds, specialists (including
attorneys) may be hired, strike funds built, and contract negotiation and implementation expenses covered.

Hospital unions in the three states clearly have some distance
to cover before they equal the number of dues checkoff clauses
negotiated by hospital unions in other parts of the United States (see
Table 5.3). On the average, twice as many hospital contracts in
Illinois, Minnesota, and Wisconsin are without dues checkoff
clauses when compared to the national hospital contract average.

TABLE 5.3

Dues Checkoff Provisions in Hospital Contracts in the
Tristate Area and the United States, 1976
(in percentages)

	Combined Tristate Contracts (N = 126)	All U.S. Hospital Contracts (N = 817)
No provision on contract	42.0	22.0
Dues checkoff	58.0	78.0

Sources: Tristate contracts: personal communication to the
authors from the Training and Employee Relations Department,
American Hospital Association. All U.S. hospital contracts:
Hervey Juris et al., "Nationwide Survey Shows Growth in Union
Contracts," Hospitals, JAHA 51 (March 16, 1977): 192.

SUMMARY: HOSPITAL BARGAINING RELATIONSHIPS

On the basis of the preceding discussion of hospital collective
bargaining relationships, a number of conclusions seem warranted.
First, the structure of labor-management relationships in the industry exhibit signs of instability. On the one hand, internal and
external pressures are forcing an increase in the size of bargaining

units, an expansion of the scope of bargaining units, and an increasing centralization of decision-making power within the bargaining structures. The tendencies of the parties themselves to engage in pattern bargaining and to encompass large numbers of union members in geographically based labor organizations are being reinforced by regulatory bodies and third-party payers.

As more and more hospitals and their employees are either incorporated into or directly affected by these centralized and expanded units, counter tendencies may appear at the grass roots level of the units to produce informal or fractional bargaining. Bargaining decisions remote from the employee may need to be interpreted loosely, or ignored entirely at times, if collective bargaining is to have relevance at individual, departmental, or occupational levels of hospitals.

The NLRB's unit policy does not seem to have been a source of fragmentation or unit proliferation, at least in Illinois, Wisconsin, and Minnesota. What fragmentation there is came into existence before 1974 and is very much restricted to Minnesota. The board, in fact, seems to be a force for expansion, rather than narrowing, of unit coverage. While it has been a focal point for criticism for some unions and most hospital representatives, the NLRB has rejected the unit policies of the state agencies and combined numerous, formerly separate occupation election units.

A key factor that would bring about further changes in bargaining structure is the relative power of labor unions in the industry to organize new workers and to generate increased bargaining leverage. Up to this point, nonnursing professional, technical, and clerical workers in the three states have remained virtually nonunion. Further, efforts by established unions in the nonprofessional as well as the nursing occupations to organize within these jurisdictions have been largely unsuccessful.

If contract provisions such as union security, dues checkoff, and wage settlements are used as a measure, the conclusion that unions have not been able to exert sufficient power to force hospitals to grant major concessions is unavoidable. (The issue of compensation and contractual constraints on manpower utilization will be examined in Chapters 7 and 8.) Should union-organizing drives prove more successful and bargaining power increase, negotiating unit expansion will likely accelerate. The norm for bargaining relationships may then be multihospital bargaining through councils or associations, perhaps on an extensive geographic basis.

NOTES

1. Neil Chamberlain, Collective Bargaining (New York: McGraw-Hill, 1951), pp. 120-58.

2. Ronald L. Miller, "The Hospital-Union Relationship—Part 1," Hospitals, JAHA 45 (May 1, 1971): 49-50.

3. Ibid., pp. 49-54.

4. Arnold R. Weber, ed., The Structure of Collective Bargaining (New York: Free Press of Glencoe, 1961), pp. xviii-xx. See especially the comments of John Dunlop, pp. 25-31.

5. Ronald L. Miller, "The Hospital Union Relationship—Part 2," Hospitals, JAHA 45 (May 16, 1971): 53.

6. Weber, Collective Bargaining, pp. 25-26.

7. See Peter Feuille, Charles Maxey, Hervey Juris, and Margaret Levi, "Determinants of Multi-Employer Bargaining in Metropolitan Hospitals," Employee Relations Law Journal 4 (Summer 1978): 98-115.

8. Based on an analysis of 126 contracts from Illinois, Minnesota, and Wisconsin supplied by the Department of Employee Relations and Training, American Hospital Association.

9. Laurence P. Corbett, "Countersaw to Whipsaw: Group Bargaining by Hospitals Meets Unions on Equal Terms" (Unpublished paper, American Hospital Association, May 1976).

10. Ibid. See also William J. Abelow and Norman Metzger, "Multi-Employer Bargaining for Health Care Institutions," Employee Relations Law Journal 1 (Winter 1976): 390-409.

11. Arthur M. Ross, Trade Union Wage Policy (Berkeley: University of California, 1948), pp. 53-64.

12. Analysis of Collective Bargaining Agreements in Chicago Area Hospitals, 1975-76 (Chicago: Chicago Hospital Council, 1975), pp. 3-21.

13. See, for example, the following for an overview of the issue of third-party payers and hospital collective bargaining: Joseph Rosmann, "Hospital Revenue Controls—Their Labor Relations and Labor Force Utilization Implications for the Hospital Industry" (Paper presented at the Thirtieth National Conference on Labor, New York University Institute of Labor Relations, May 17, 1977); and Carl J. Schramm, "Continuing Hospital Labor Costs—A Separate-Industries Approach," Employee Relations Law Journal 4 (Summer 1978): 82-97.

14. Information obtained from an analysis of 126 hospital collective bargaining contracts supplied to the authors by the Training and Employee Relations Department of the American Hospital Association.

15. Hervey Juris et al., "Nationwide Survey Shows Growth in Union Contracts," Hospitals, JAHA 51 (March 16, 1977): 192.

16. See Juris et al., "Growth in Union Contracts," pp. 128, 130.

6

LABOR-MANAGEMENT CONFLICT IN HOSPITALS: EXTENT, SOURCES, AND RESOLUTION

The inevitability of labor-management conflict in hospitals as a consequence of unionization was one of the most seriously discussed issues during the congressional hearings on the 1974 health-care amendments. Many speakers noted that because hospitals were different from industrial enterprises (in that alternative sources of health care may be limited and hospital services cannot be stockpiled) their services must be provided on a continuous basis.[1] The immediate impact of an interruption in health care, it was argued, could fall on the patient with perhaps disastrous results.

> [An] extremely high price will be exacted if strikes
> occur in the hospital setting. Not an economic cost,
> but a human cost. The human cost of suffering or
> loss of life. The human cost resulting from an inabil-
> ity to restore vital life functions because of delay in
> bringing appropriate [sic] skills to bear. A second, a
> minute, an hour, a day—each of these can be the criti-
> cal time span which determines success or failure in
> treatment of a sick or injured person.[2]

As Dennis Pointer observed, many on the management side saw the mere recognition of unions as an invitation to strikes.[3]

From an empirical standpoint, it is not clear exactly how much conflict occurs, in what form it becomes manifest, what impact it has on hospitals, or how efficient existing forms of dispute resolution are.[4] Case studies made during the course of hospital work stoppages seem to indicate that labor disputes may not be as disastrous for hospitals as might be supposed. Strikes may be short, patients transferred, elective surgery postponed, picket lines opened for deliveries, employee vacancies covered with personnel reassignments and volunteers, and so forth.[5]

Further, the forms in which the disputes take place may have different implications for hospitals than for conventional industrial enterprises. Thus, although picketing may be a formidable weapon, such devices as secondary boycotts, particularly of the consumer variety, seem to have little relevance. In addition, as is generally true in the public sector, the withholding of labor may surface as slowdowns, "sickouts," "nurse-ins," mass resignations, and work-to-rule, among others.

In examining the amount and impact of labor conflict in the hospitals of Illinois, Minnesota, and Wisconsin, those disputes associated with union organizing and contract negotiation will be considered first. Included will be a discussion of the mechanisms for their resolution, provided either by law or by the parties themselves. Second, we will review the experience of hospital labor and management with disputes that arise over the interpretation of existing contracts or, as they are customarily labeled, "rights" disputes. To the extent possible, relevant comparisons will be made with experience in the general hospital or health-care industry in the United States and with non-health-care sectors.

DISPUTES

Recognition

A recurring argument made by witnesses at hearings on the health-care amendments, held from 1971 to 1973, was that much of the labor conflict present in the hospital industry up to that time arose from a lack of machinery to resolve disputes over union demands for recognition. Support for this argument comes from the data in Table 6.1, which show that of 248 health-care work stoppages in the private sector recorded by the U.S. Department of Labor for the period 1962 to 1972, slightly more than 50 percent (125) were associated with efforts to achieve recognition. Witnesses also pointed out that the incidence of such strikes was much less in those states in which organizing rights were protected and representation election machinery was available. For those states that had no machinery, inclusion of the industry under federal labor law would fill the gap by providing an appropriate system for dealing with organizing disputes.

Experience in the three states under examination here supports the position of those who favored expansion of the federal jurisdiction. In Wisconsin and Minnesota, where state labor boards supplied forums for handling disputes over recognition, no strikes of this kind occurred in either private or public sector hospitals through 1974. In Illinois, on the other hand, which lacked a comparable legal framework, there were a number of strikes for recognition, first by AFSCME and then by HELP in the 1960s. Ultimately, the explosiveness of the situation led the parties to devise their own machinery—the so-called preelection agreements. Subsequently, these ad hoc procedures were used in more than 30 elections.

TABLE 6.1

Work Stoppages in the Health-Care Industry (SIC 80)
by Sector and Cause

	Private Sector			Government Sector		
	Recognition	Other	Total	Recognition	Other	Total
1962	2	4	6	*	*	*
1963	7	6	13	1	0	1
1964	6	8	14	*	*	*
1965	8	5	13	1	0	1
1966	9	10	19	2	16	18
1967	14	13	27	7	12	19
1968	14	14	28	4	17	21
1969	21	22	43	5	17	22
1970	26	23	49	6	20	26
1971	18	18	36	4	14	18
Total	125	123	248	30	96	126

*Data not available.
Source: U.S., Department of Labor, Bureau of Labor Statistics, personal communication to the authors.

Unions in the private sector of Illinois were free to employ coercion in the form of strikes, picketing, and demonstrations where persuasion failed. In contrast, unions attempting to organize hospitals in the public sector were subject to court ordered injunctions if work stoppages occurred. Yet the record reveals that 28 strikes did occur from 1966 to 1974 in the state's public health institutions, and that approximately 36 percent were a consequence of recognition disputes.[6] With no alternatives available, employees will engage in strikes or related activities even if they are illegal.

Negotiation

In Minnesota and Wisconsin, there have been almost no labor disputes on the private hospital scene from the late 1940s to 1976. Conflict in Minnesota hospitals in the mid-1940s led to the passage of the Charitable Hospitals Act, and from that time to the advent of federal jurisdiction only one stoppage occurred.[7] The absence of open warfare was typical of nursing homes and of public health-care institutions in which strikes played a very minimal role in labor relations (see Table 6.2).

Wisconsin's record in its private sector hospitals nearly equals that of Minnesota. Apparently, no strikes occurred before 1969[8] and only four since. As the table indicates, the incidence of strikes among other private and public health-care institutions (13 work stoppages having taken place between 1966 and 1975) is considerably greater than that of the private, nonprofit hospitals. It should be noted that the six public sector strikes were in violation of the state's prohibition on such activity.

Illinois has by far the worst strike record for the three states, recording more work stoppages in all categories of health institutions. It is of interest to observe that, despite the illegality of public employee strikes, state and local health-care institutions experienced more strikes than their counterparts in the private sector.

Finally, concerning the incidence of strikes, Table 6.2 indicates that of the 68 total stoppages that have occurred in the 1966 to 1975 decade, only 18 (26 percent) involved private, nonprofit hospitals. When one considers that in the three states combined there are approximately 150 bargaining units covered by labor agreements in nonprofit hospitals, it is clear that recognition of a union is not an invitation to strike. On the contrary, the amount of labor peace is quite remarkable.

Duration of Strikes

An additional dimension of labor disputes, beyond the sheer number of strikes, is how long they last. One observer contended that hospital strikes during the 1960s generally were short, lasting six days on the average, and that this brevity tended to strengthen a union's bargaining power. "Given the short time duration of the strike action and the pressures to resume 'production,' the hospital's cost of disagreement with the union's terms is considerably greater than the union's cost of disagreement with the management's terms."[9] The generalization that "management cannot win strikes of short duration" was believed by the observer to be particularly relevant for the hospital industry.

TABLE 6.2

Work Stoppages in the Health-Care Industry in Illinois, Minnesota, and Wisconsin

	Illinois				Wisconsin				Minnesota				Combined Total
	Private Hospital	Private Nursing Homes	Government Hospitals and Nursing Homes	Total	Private Hospital	Private Nursing Homes	Government Hospitals and Nursing Homes	Total	Private Hospital	Private Nursing Homes	Government Hospitals and Nursing Homes	Total	
1966	0	0	2	2	0	0	2	2	0	1	0	1	5
1967	2	0	3	5	0	0	0	0	0	0	0	0	5
1968	0	0	3	3	0	0	0	0	0	0	0	0	3
1969	3	1	5	9	1	0	0	1	0	0	0	0	10
1970	0	2	4	6	0	1	2	3	0	0	0	0	9
1971	2	1	3	6	0	1	1	2	0	0	0	0	8
1972	2	1	2	5	1	3	0	4	0	0	0	0	9
1973	3	0	2	5	1	0	0	1	0	0	0	0	6
1974	1	3	1	5	1	1	0	2	0	0	0	0	7
1975	1	2	0	3	0	1	1	2	0	1	0	1	6
Total	14	10	25	49	4	7	6	17	0	2	0	2	68

Source: U.S., Department of Labor, Bureau of Labor Statistics, personal communication to the authors.

The short duration of hospital strikes in the decade of the 1960s contrasted markedly with that for industry generally. Data from the Bureau of Labor Statistics indicate that over the years 1961 to 1969, the average strike in industry lasted 23.5 days, nearly four times longer than those in hospitals.[10] The logic of the argument suggests that hospital unions are much more powerful than their industrial counterparts. However, this conclusion needs to be examined more completely before it can be accepted.

In Table 6.3, the average duration of strikes for health-care institutions in the three states is compared with the equivalent figure for all U.S. industries, by type of institution. The average of 21 days on strike for private hospitals is not very different from the 24-day figure for all U.S. industries. The mean for government institutions (25) is even closer to the U.S. average. Finally, for reasons unknown to the investigators, the average days on strike is much greater for private nursing homes and related health-care institutions than for private, profit and nonprofit hospitals, suggesting that the private health-care industry should not be treated as a homogeneous unit, but that its data should be disaggregated by the appropriate three-digit Standard Industrial Classifications (SIC).

TABLE 6.3

Mean Number of Days on Strike in the Tristate Health-Care Industry, and in All U.S. Industries, 1966-75

U.S.		Combined Tristate Data	
All Industries	Private Hospitals	Nursing Homes and Others	Government Hospitals and Nursing Homes
24.34	21.23	32.50	25.26

Note: For private hospitals, range = 1-73 days; for nursing homes, 1-127; for government hospitals, 2-127.

Source: Calculated from data supplied by the U.S. Bureau of Labor Statistics, Office of Wages and Industrial Relations.

Distribution of strikes by year of occurrence does not reveal a trend toward either longer or shorter strikes. The length of work stoppages varied randomly over the ten-year period. In addition, the combined data for the three states are obviously considerably in excess of the average of six days that others associate with the hospital industry during the 1960s.[11] It is difficult to explain why the discrepancy should be so great between the strike experience of Minnesota, Wisconsin, and Illinois and that of hospitals in the United States generally during that period.

A possible explanation is that the nature of the strikes was different. Minnesota, Wisconsin, and Illinois had formal mechanisms for handling recognition disputes (the latter by action of the parties). Thus, the work stoppage for recognition, which was so prevalent generally in the United States before 1974, was unnecessary in any of the three states. It is also possible that the health-care unions in the area lack the bargaining power of their counterparts elsewhere in the United States, and that the longer average duration of hospital strikes is a reflection of this.

Number of Workers on Strike

The prospect of thousands of workers simultaneously walking out of a community's hospitals is grim. Although Congress stopped short of prohibiting hospital work stoppages entirely, it did provide for a number of mediation and "cooling off" periods along with the mechanism of the boards of inquiry to forestall such an eventuality. That such potentially calamitous disputes can be a reality was demonstrated in hospital strikes in the San Francisco Bay Area and most notably in New York City, where a work stoppage in 1976 involved more than 40,000 workers.[12]

The potential for such strikes exists also in the tristate area. Bargaining units in Minnesota may cover upwards of 20 hospitals and more than 5,000 workers. In Illinois, although negotiating units are smaller, one Chicago union, HELP, tends to control most of the city's nonprofessional hospital workers. Although the potential is less in Wisconsin, where unionization is more uneven in urban areas and across government and nonprofit hospitals, there, too, negotiation units may approach 1,000 employees, a not inconsequential number.

A review of strikes in the three states reveals that Minnesota, where the consequences would be the worst, has had no strikes of private hospitals since 1956. Wisconsin has had only four work stoppages in nearly 30 years of hospital bargaining. If there is currently a strike problem, it would have to be in Illinois.

Since 1966, Illinois has had 14 private hospital strikes involving a total of 1,115 workers. The largest unit was composed of 174 employees who stayed off the job one day. The mean number of workers involved in hospital strikes in Illinois is 79.6; in Wisconsin it is 53.3.[13]

The record does not support the premise that hospital recognition of unions is an invitation to strike. By almost any measure, the health-care labor scene has been peaceful with rare exceptions. Moreover, the procedures for dispute settlement established under the 1974 amendments have very likely further reduced the possibilities for conflict. Recognition is no longer an issue for strikes, extended warning and mediation periods have been provided, and, if all else fails, the board of inquiry can be invoked before a stoppage occurs.

It is not appropriate to project this sense of health-care tranquillity too far into the future. Hospitals and negotiating units are growing larger, and cost containment issues are beginning to intrude on the bargaining. Should the union leadership become more militant and the unions themselves stronger, the bargaining relationships could deteriorate into the more combative stances now characteristic of the East and West Coast hospital sectors. Neither historical harmony nor government strategies for resolving disputes may prevent wholesale disruption in the operation of the hospitals in the three states.

RESOLUTION OF NEGOTIATION DISPUTES

Pre-1974

Procedures for resolving new contract disputes varied considerably among the three states before they came under federal jurisdiction. Wisconsin did not differentiate between classes of private employees, permitting all to picket and strike without constraints. The maximum form of state intervention was mediation supplied by the Wisconsin Employee Relations Commission.

In the public sector, state and local government employers were presumably under the WERC, but without statutory guidelines until 1959 when the Municipal Employment Relations Act was passed. The MERA was later supplemented by the State Employment Labor Relations Act of 1966 and in 1972 to 1973 by a statute that provided for arbitration of impasses involving fire fighters and police officers, except those in the city of Milwaukee.[14] In addition, the municipal law itself was amended in 1978 to provide for the right to strike if both labor and management decline to arbitrate their disputes.

Either by statute or voluntary agreement, arbitration of hospital negotiation disputes became an important element in collective bargaining in both Minnesota and Illinois. An examination of health-care labor relations in Wisconsin, however, reveals no recorded cases of interest arbitration in hospital labor disputes. Agreements were reached through bargaining without resort to strike before 1969, and in all save a few instances since then.

In Minnesota, both public and private hospitals were subject to the Charitable Hospitals Act, which not only banned strikes but also required arbitration of all impasses over "interests" or "rights." The CHA stipulated that arbitration could be initiated by either party to the dispute; a three-person arbitration panel was to be constituted by having each party appoint one member who then would be joined by a neutral designated by the governor;[†] and all strikes, lockouts, and picketing were subject to court injunction. Matters of union security were not considered arbitrable under the law. Also excluded were issues related to the "internal management of hospitals."

Measured by the objective of securing labor peace in hospitals, the CHA was an unqualified success. Strikes and picketing virtually disappeared from the Minnesota hospital scene after 1947.[15] By other criteria success seems to be less clear cut. From 1947 to 1969, one of the major unions, SEIU Local 113, had arbitrated all but one of its contracts in Minneapolis-St. Paul. The Minnesota Nurses Association also resorted to third-party resolution on a number of occasions. By 1962 the system had been invoked at least 15 times, half of those by the same union.[16]

The prospect that compulsory interest arbitration will have a "narcotic" effect or that it will tend to "chill" collective bargaining in good faith has long been cited as a rationale against requiring it in conflict resolution. Although there is no consensus, a number of individuals maintain that the CHA's stipulation that all hospital labor disputes be arbitrated did indeed cast a chill over collective bargaining.[17] Some individuals who had firsthand experience with the law felt that the parties tended to freeze their positions even before a formal petition for arbitration was submitted. In addition, the mechanism apparently was often used for internal political reasons. In an interview published in 1965, the then Assistant State Labor Conciliator Vern Buck argued:

> Both management and labor could shoulder more responsibility and settle more cases in conciliation, and would do so if compulsory arbitration were not available. . . . It is far easier to go to his membership, and say "look what we got stuck with due to that

---

[†]Following amendments to the CHA in 1969, the governor no longer appointed the neutral. Instead the members designated by the parties to the arbitration panel selected the neutral.

no-good arbitrator" than work face to face with the
other side to gain an equitable settlement which they
would have to justify to their boards or membership. [18]

Further, after years of arbitration, contracts tended to become "a cumbersome accumulation of arbitrated provisions" which
the parties had little success in clarifying through direct negotiations. [19] By the late 1960s, "the compulsory arbitration law [had]
become a shelter for poor labor relations practices between the
parties." [20]

Notwithstanding the Charitable Hospitals Act, what some
people describe as the "excessive" use of arbitration did achieve
important results in eliminating labor strife in hospitals. In addition, it also had important consequences for bargaining outcomes
throughout the state. The custom of pattern bargaining in Minnesota,
in which the key settlements were those of the registered nurses of
the MNA and the nonprofessional Service Employees of Local 113 in
Minneapolis-St. Paul, meant that the arbitration awards provided
the bench marks for negotiations throughout the state. Large hospitals in such cities as Rochester and Duluth, among others, took
their cues directly from the arbitrators' awards. Moreover, the
impact was felt not only by unionized but by nonunionized employees
as well. Thus, although the arbitration mechanism of the CHA was
rarely employed outside the Twin Cities, it had a profound effect
elsewhere.

Finally, it should be pointed out that by the mid-1960s, Minnesota hospital employees were no longer among the wage leaders for
the industry in the United States. Arbitration did not result in large
wage increases; in fact, awards and settlements were quite conservative. [21] It is of interest that despite a relative decline in their
income compared to hospital employees in areas where strikes,
legal or otherwise, were still a major factor in bargaining, the at-
tachment to interest arbitration continued on a voluntary basis in
Minnesota after 1974.

Illinois, and particularly Chicago, was a scene of much hospital labor conflict in the 1960s, and the absence of a state legal
framework by which either disputes could be resolved or strikes
and picketing prohibited compelled the parties to devise their own
systems. Thus, the so-called preelection agreement was born in
agreements between HELP and certain Chicago hospitals. [22] In
addition to describing the bargaining unit and the machinery by which
the election would be held, a no-strike-no-lockout clause was included that applied to both contract application and negotiation disputes.

Although the arbitration clauses existed in most of the pre-election agreements created, apparently they were invoked only once before 1974 and twice between 1974 and 1977. The clauses' importance, however, rested with the union's willingness to forgo strikes in exchange for the right to take disputes to a neutral third party should an impasse occur. As will be discussed below, the parties continue to honor the preelection agreements even though they are now of questionable enforceability.

Post-1974

Anxiety over the consequences of disputes in hospitals and other health-care facilities persuaded Congress to include unique dispute settlement procedures in the amendment that deleted the charitable hospital exclusion from the Taft-Hartley Act. Mandatory mediation was prescribed, and prior notification of intent to change contracts was required far in advance of any negotiations. The rights to strike and picket were protected, but were allowed only after a ten-day warning was given to the targeted hospital. These procedures were intended not only to enable government mediators to have time to find ways to get the parties together before a work stoppage occurred, but also, once a strike was threatened, to generate pressures from the community to push the parties toward a settlement.[23] Should a strike eventuate, the ten-day warning would give hospital administrators an opportunity to carry out activities necessary for the safety and well-being of patients, including their transfer to other hospitals.

Finally, if, in the opinion of the director of the Federal Mediation and Conciliation Service, a strike would "substantially interrupt the delivery of health care in the locality concerned," a board of inquiry could be established to investigate the issues and make a written report to the parties.[24] A BOI was to be appointed 30 days after FMCS received its notice from the parties and was required to report 15 days before the contract expired.

Disagreements between health employers and the service have arisen over the interpretation of the time frame provided in the law for appointing the BOIs.[25] FMCS argues that it can wait until 30 days before the contract expires to create a BOI. Some employers contend that if a BOI is to be set up, the service must do so within 30 days after it has been notified by one of the parties of an intent to change an agreement, even if this notification has been made far in advance of the 60-day requirement set by the law. The issue is now before the courts for final determination.

The FMCS was prone to appoint boards of inquiry much more frequently during the first year of the amendments than thereafter. In the first four months alone, 24 BOIs were established.[26] An additional 31 BOIs were named between January and July 1975. Through the end of July 1977, 50 more had been established; 37 in 1976-77; and 34 more for the 12 months ending in August 1978.[27]

The board of inquiry has not been a factor in the settlement of hospital labor disputes in the three states under investigation here. As of February 1978, only seven BOIs had been appointed for the entire region in the period since August 1974. This is in contrast to other regions of the United States, notably the Northeast and West Coast, where the FMCS's case load and the number of BOI appointments have been much higher.[28]

For several reasons, it is not surprising that FMCS has found little reason to invoke the BOI section of the Taft-Hartley amendments. First, there have been few bargaining impasses in which strikes were threatened in any of the three states. Second, the negotiating structure and extent of unionism, particularly in Illinois and Wisconsin, are such that substantial interruptions to the delivery of health care are not likely to occur. Finally, the parties in Minneapolis-St. Paul and Chicago, the two major centers of hospital union activity in their respective states, have made provisions in many of their contracts to employ binding arbitration should negotiations break down.

The last point needs further discussion given the framework for dispute settlement that existed in Illinois and Minnesota prior to 1974. In the former case, the preelection agreements constrained the use of concerted action by the major union involved, HELP, and imposed arbitration for bargaining impasses. Although it is conceivable that these agreements are no longer binding, the parties have chosen, in most situations, to continue to respect them.[29] Thus, for example, two cases involving new contract issues have gone to arbitration since the 1974 amendments.

The parties in Minnesota, especially those covered by HMMI contracts, have also seen fit to continue with a system of no-strike binding arbitration of negotiation impasses. When the CHA was preempted by federal law, agreements to arbitrate interest disputes for up to ten years were made between Health Manpower Management and the Minnesota Nurses Association, Local 113 of the SEIU, and most, although not all, of the other unions bargaining with Twin Cities hospitals. Illustrative is the pertinent clause from the MNA contract that covers the period June 1, 1974, through May 31, 1980.

> In the event the parties are unable to agree by negotia-
> tion on the terms of succeeding agreements to replace,

modify or change any contract agreement expiring or reopening prior to May 31, 1980, the provisions of the succeeding contract agreement shall be determined by arbitration as provided in this Section 20. Either party may submit the unresolved issues to arbitration by written notice to the other party. [30]

The clause further provides for a three-member board in which each of the parties, following the former CHA requirements, designates an arbitrator, who in turn select the third. Arbitration issues are to be decided by the board of arbitration within the general boundaries of "unresolved issues with respect to 'wages, hours, and other terms and conditions of employment.'" In this regard, the scope of arbitration is now considerably wider than it was under the Charitable Hospitals Act in which items dealing with union security and internal hospital management were excluded.

In addition, a few labor-management relationships outside the Twin Cities are also resorting to arbitration of negotiation disputes. In Rochester two of the hospitals associated with the Mayo Clinic have used neutrals for such disputes in recent years. The process does not seem to have been built into the contracts but is being used on an ad hoc and voluntary basis.

In Wisconsin, no trends have appeared suggesting increased use of interest arbitration either contractually or ad hoc. The parties seem to have shunned the use of neutrals in negotiating disputes, reserving, although not often using, the right to strike when impasses are reached.

The general tendency across the three states is to not build agreements to arbitrate negotiation impasses into labor contracts. Keeping in mind that in the Twin Cities single contracts cover up to 23 hospitals and that in Chicago the preelection agreements are separate from the regular labor contracts, the practice of the parties is to not bind themselves to arbitrate "interests." An examination of 126 hospital contracts for the tristate area shows that only 15 percent have such clauses. [31] Further, this category of arbitration clauses provides virtually no limitations on the arbitrator and no criteria to guide his award. Finally, the newer innovations in third-party resolution, including "med-arb" and final-offer arbitration, are entirely absent.

GRIEVANCE DISPUTES

Contrary to the situation with "interest" arbitration, clauses requiring the arbitration of disputes over the interpretation or application of existing contracts are almost universal in hospital labor agreements in the three states. Only 2.4 percent of 126 hospital contracts examined for the area lack grievance procedures, and only 2 percent of the contracts have grievance procedures that do not terminate in binding arbitration.[32] Nonunion hospitals also frequently provide grievance procedures, usually without arbitration as the final step.

As shown in Table 6.4, nearly two-thirds of the contracts in the three states have only three steps, including arbitration. Most of the remaining third have only one additional step. This pattern contrasts significantly with the grievance procedures in hospital contracts in other parts of the United States in which, on the average, only half as many contain three steps and a much greater proportion have as many as five and six steps.

TABLE 6.4

Distribution of Hospital Union Contracts by Number of Steps in the Formal Grievance Procedure, 1976 (in percentages)

Number of Steps in Grievance Procedure	Tristate Contracts (N = 126)	All U.S. Hospital Contracts (N = 817)
No provision	2.4	2.9
1	0.0	0.4
2	22.2	7.8
3	36.5	20.4
4	31.7	46.5
5	6.3	18.1
6	0.8	2.4
7	0.0	0.1
Other	0.0	1.2

Sources: Tristate contracts: Division of Employee Relations and Training, American Hospital Association, personal communication to the authors; U.S. contracts: Hervey Juris et al., "Employer Discipline No Longer Management Prerogative Only," Hospitals, JAHA 51 (May 1, 1977): 71.

Typically, the first step involves the employee and a supervisor. The hospital personnel director comes in at the second step, and the hospital administrator at the third step, if it is used. Arbitration is the final step.

Although certain subjects may be contractually excluded from the grievance machinery and arbitration, as were internal hospital management and union security under the Charitable Hospitals Act in Minnesota, collective contracts in Illinois, Minnesota, and Wisconsin rarely contain such provisions. In Table 6.5, we see that no mention is made of union security, and insignificant numbers of contracts exclude hospital administration. When the tristate contracts are compared with those reviewed in Juris's general survey, there is some evidence that grievance procedures and arbitration are narrower in scope than in other geographical regions, particularly those concerning hospital administration issues.

TABLE 6.5

Distribution of Subjects Excluded from Grievance and
Arbitration Procedures in Tristate and
U.S. Hospitals, 1976
(in percentage of contracts)

	Grievance		Arbitration	
Excluded Subject	Tristate Hospitals (N = 126)	All Private U.S. Hospitals (N = 512)	Tristate Hospitals (N = 126)	All Private U.S. Hospitals (N = 512)
Wages	0.8	2.5	5.6	7.8
Hospital administration	0.8	6.3	2.4	12.9
Supplementary benefits	0.8	3.5	0.8	4.9
Job security	0.0	0.0	0.0	0.0
Other	9.5	9.8	12.7	10.5

Sources: Tristate data: Division of Employee Relations and Training, American Hospital Association, personal communication to the authors; all U.S. hospitals: Hervey Juris et al., "Employee Discipline No Longer Management Prerogative Only," Hospitals, JAHA 51 (May 1, 1977): 71.

In recent years, grievance and arbitration procedures have come to be looked on generally as a quid pro quo for the no-strike clause. It is useful to note, therefore, that in hospital contracts in the three states, no-strike clauses are far less prevalent than grievance or arbitration clauses. Of 126 contracts analyzed, 46 percent lacked such a clause. [33] Where it did appear, however, the ban was absolute. General U.S. hospital contract data analyzed by the Juris group indicate that 75 percent of the hospitals "had some type of no-strike provision." [34]

In Minnesota contracts, the lack of a no-strike ban is understandable. Since the CHA prohibited all hospital strikes for whatever reason, stipulating compulsory arbitration to resolve both negotiation and grievance disputes, before 1974 it would have been redundant to place such clauses in hospital labor contracts. On the other hand, it is not clear why the frequency of such clauses should be so low in the other two states, particularly when the general hospital industry practice is to incorporate them in agreements.

Although rights or obligations may be contractually stated, in fact the provisions may not be resorted to in the manner or frequency that the parties anticipated when a collective agreement was negotiated. This seems to be the case with the grievance and arbitration clauses of the hospital contracts in the three states. Data compiled from the mailed questionnaires and field interviews suggest that despite their availability, the grievance machinery is used infrequently and resort to arbitration is almost nonexistent. On the average, less than one case per year per hospital was taken to arbitration. In general, the most frequent issue to be grieved is the scheduling of employees' hours and particularly weekends off.

Hospitals operate continuously around the clock; thus, night shifts and work on weekends and holidays are the rule. The problems of satisfying employee needs for normal working days and time off to spend holidays with family or friends become acute. These are issues often raised in negotiations and, if not satisfactorily resolved, labor or management may attempt to persuade an arbitrator to give, through an award, what was not obtained at the bargaining table.

While it may be argued that on some occasions grievance and arbitration systems were misused for political purposes, this practice seems to be the exception rather than the rule. In fact, if one uses the number of grievances filed and the proportion of them ultimately carried to arbitration as criteria of conflict, the conclusion would follow that the level of labor-management disputes within hospitals is low in the tristate area. This finding is also consistent with other measures of conflict, such as work stoppages, which give low readings of frequency or severity of disputes between the parties, and with the conclusions of other authors studying labor-management conflict in hospitals in other regions of the United States.[35]

LABOR-MANAGEMENT CONFLICT IN HOSPITALS: SOME CONCLUDING THOUGHTS

Although collective bargaining disputes in such cities as New York and San Francisco are highly publicized, such conflict is not representative of hospital collective bargaining generally in the United States.[36] It is also not consistent with the tristate area in which labor-management conflict in the hospital industry has been minimal and close to the national average. It is appropriate at this point, therefore, to examine more closely the relative absence of conflict so that this particular dimension of labor relations in hospitals can be understood more fully. While such explanations may not be readily generalized beyond Illinois, Minnesota, and Wisconsin, they may nevertheless enable us to know, for this area at least, why there was so little conflict in the past and whether the situation will change in the future.

It is often observed in industrial relations that the older and more mature the bargaining relationship, the less likely conflict will occur. If it is assumed that this statement is true, it would be useful to inquire into the maturity of hospital bargaining relationships in the three states that were the object of our research. One finds that despite the fact that federal collective bargaining legislation is recent for the health-care industry, the parties have been bargaining for many years in Minnesota, Wisconsin, and Illinois hospitals. Minnesota nurses had 50 bargaining units by 1948,[37] only a few short of the number in 1978. The SEIU also has represented service workers in major hospital bargaining units in Minnesota for approximately 30 years. In fact, nearly all of the hospital bargaining relationships are long established, whether within the Twin Cities, out of state, or across professional and nonprofessional employee levels.

In Wisconsin, the first nonprofit hospital bargaining unit was recognized in 1941, and by June 30, 1968, 35 had been established.[38] The mean age of the 39 formal bargaining units in existence in 1977 is 11 years.

In contrast, the average bargaining unit in Illinois is only about six and a half years old. Thus, given the fact that labor-management conflict has been highest in Illinois hospitals, lowest in Minnesota, and at an intermediate point in Wisconsin, age of the relationship appears closely associated with level of conflict.

Other factors also have contributed to the rarity of labor disputes in the industry. First, the long period of time that the parties in Minnesota had to adjust to each other was, for the most part, within the context of the Charitable Hospitals Act. Twenty-seven years of no strikes and compulsory arbitration have thoroughly conditioned both sides to accept this approach as workable and potential settlements as fair.

Belief in "Nightingaleism," that is, in service to patients before personal needs,[39] and fear of the consequences of hospital stoppages also continue to be strong motivational factors. Under such circumstances, it is not surprising that, contrary to the unions' customary bargaining position that the right to strike must never be abridged, more peaceful means of conflict resolution are positively perceived.[40]

Minnesota constitutes a prime example of the impact the social system can have on the bargaining behavior of participants in an industrial relations system. Its labor force, including managers, professionals, and unskilled workers, is largely middle class, well educated, and drawn from similar ethnic and racial backgrounds. Thus, the social or class conflicts that may spill over into the hospitals in other areas of the United States are, for the most part, not a factor in Minnesota health-care labor relations. This generalization is also true for most of Wisconsin and downstate Illinois. The hospital labor force of Milwaukee constitutes a partial exception and, of course, the nonprofessional workers in Chicago clearly do not fit the generalization.

Beyond the particular attitude or beliefs that may be associated with the citizens of a state or community, other demographic, personal, or job-related characteristics of the population may affect the amount and form of conflict that occurs. These characteristics may either reinforce or reduce an individual's propensity to engage in conflict.[41] In the case of hospital workers, these characteristics presently seem to contribute to the reduction of conflict, even in such cities as Chicago or Milwaukee where social or ethnic differences would otherwise elevate tensions in the workplace. First, the labor force tends to be a floating one, with very high rates of mobility even among professional workers. With high rates of turnover, building a strong membership base is difficult for a union. Finances may be weak and loyalties to the union not well developed. Employees who are unhappy with their work situation may leave to look for better work rather than stay on the job in hopes that a union can bring improvement.

Second, large numbers of hospital employees are young females who may see themselves as only temporary members of the labor force and, therefore, as having little to gain from an investment in union building and collective bargaining. Given the gradual change in the labor market behavior of women, these beliefs also may be altered so that long-term organizational and professional commitments assume higher priorities.

The high proportion of females in hospitals tends to dampen conflict in another way as well. General social values that stress female passiveness toward, subservience to, and complementarity (not competitiveness) with males place a premium on obedience to the predominantly male medical staff and administrators of the typical hospital. Joining unions (as opposed to associations), haggling over wages, picketing, and striking raise negative connotations of aggressive, greedy, unladylike, and, therefore, unacceptable behavior by female employees.[42]

Under the above circumstances, one would not expect to find strong labor organizations led by militant union officers. Leaders have been militant in the nonprofessional organizations for periods of time—Local 113 in the Twin Cities until the 1960s and HELP in its formative period in Chicago. The trend, however, is away from militancy toward accommodation and cooperation rather than conflict. Critics argue that such unions as HELP are remiss in not placing greater stress on civil rights issues to stimulate greater solidarity and militancy among their members in the manner of District 1199 in New York.[43] Perhaps with the new federal amendments attitudes and behavior of both union leaders and members will become more aggressive. In the meantime, trade union behavior in the three states will likely continue to be one of consolidation of past gains and maintenance of the status quo without a high level of grievances or bargaining impasses.

Finally, a major influence on the industrial relations climate is the attitude and behavior of hospital managers. Strenuous efforts are being made to counter union-organizing drives and to resolve employee problems quickly. Administrators with labor relations experience are being hired, grievance procedures even in nonunion hospitals are being created, personnel supervisors are being sent to labor relations seminars, and consultants are being retained to advise and represent the hospital on union-related issues. In general, the personnel function is being greatly expanded and updated, often at the expense of other functional areas.

In addition, the practice of granting salary and benefit increases achieved in bargaining to nonunion employees in unionized or nonunion hospitals is widespread. Labeled as the "threat effect," this policy may result in compensation levels in the nonunion sector that not only equal but in fact may exceed those of the unionized hospital sector. Thus, sources of conflict and employee dissatisfaction may be effectively removed.

NOTES

1. See, for example, U.S., Congress, Senate, Subcommittee
on Labor of the Committee on Labor and Public Welfare, Coverage
of Nonprofit Hospitals under National Labor Relations Act, 1973:
Hearings on S. 794 and S. 2292, 93rd Cong., 1st sess., July 31,
August 1, 2, and October 4, 1973, pp. 158-285.

2. Ibid., p. 165.

3. Dennis D. Pointer, Unionization, Collective Bargaining,
and the Non-Profit Hospital, Center for Labor and Management
Monograph Series no. 13 (Iowa City: University of Iowa, 1969),
p. 19.

4. See Senate, Hearings on S. 794 and S. 2292, p. 233.
There was some confusion at the hearings because of discrepancies
in hospital strike data supplied to the Subcommittee not only by the
witnesses but also the U.S. Department of Labor as well.

5. See Pointer, Unionization, p. 32.

6. Personal communication to investigators, U.S. Bureau of
Labor Statistics, Office of Wages and Industrial Relations, March
17, 1977.

7. Ronald L. Miller, "Collective Bargaining in Non-Profit
Hospitals" (Ph.D. diss., University of Pennsylvania, 1969), p. 237.

8. Pointer, Unionization, pp. 34-35.

9. Ibid., p. 25.

10. U.S., Department of Labor, Bureau of Labor Statistics,
Handbook of Labor Statistics (Washington, D.C.: Government
Printing Office, 1975), p. 390, table 159.

11. Pointer, Unionization, pp. 34-35.

12. Bureau of National Affairs, Daily Labor Report no. 18
(January 26, 1977), pp. 3-13.

13. Calculated by data provided by the U.S. Bureau of Labor
Statistics, Office of Wages and Industrial Relations.

14. For a detailed discussion of the Wisconsin police and fire
arbitration law, see James L. Stern et al., Final Offer Arbitration
(Lexington, Mass.: D. C. Heath, 1975).

15. See Duane R. Carlson, "Minnesota's Pioneer Hospital
Labor Act: Model or Mistake?," Modern Hospital 104 (May 1965):
106-10. One of the few strikes of record occurred in Children's
Hospital of St. Paul during the fall of 1964. Stemming from a dispute over the work schedules of housekeeping and kitchen employees,
which had been unilaterally changed by the hospital management,
Local 113 of the SEIU called a work stoppage in protest and set up
a picket line. The strike was enjoined under the CHA after two days
of picketing and the dispute then submitted to arbitration.

16. New York State, Joint Legislative Committee on Industrial and Labor Conditions, "Binding Arbitration in Minnesota Hospitals," in Report 1962-63, Legislative Document, 1963, no. 38, pp. 68-69.

17. For a major dissent to this point see New York State, "Binding Arbitration," p. 70. This paper, prepared for the New York state legislature in 1962, found the CHA "to be a sound instrument of public policy. It has kept the hospitals free from the dread of work stoppages. It has promoted equitable working standards for hospital employees. And, for the most part, it has accomplished these ends without crippling collective bargaining." See also the evaluation of the CHA offered at the House Hearings on H.R. 13678 held in 1974 that reached the same conclusion: U.S., Congress, House, Coverage of Nonprofit Hospitals under the National Labor Relations Act: Report Together with Additional Views, 93rd Cong., 2d sess., May 20, 1974, pp. 15-16.

18. Carlson, "Minnesota's Pioneer Hospital Labor Act," p. 108.

19. Miller, "Collective Bargaining," p. 238.

20. Ibid.

21. Ibid., p. 169, table 15.

22. Ibid., pp. 308-12 for an example of one such preelection agreement.

23. For example, Richard F. Schubert, Under Secretary of Labor in 1973, in reviewing the justification for the ten-day strike notice commented, "I think our primary objective was to bring all the forces available in the public to bear on the parties. In other words, obviously, the mayors of the communities, in some cases the governors of the states, responsible officials, health organizations on a local basis and on a state basis, would be involved in the 10-day period to maximize the pressure, again, on the parties, to come to some kind of realistic resolution." Hearings, May 20, 1974, p. 436.

24. Public Law 93-360, section 213.

25. See Bureau of National Affairs, Daily Labor Report, no. 88 (May 5, 1977), pp. A14 and A15.

26. James F. Scearce and Lucretia Dewey Tanner, "Health Care Bargaining: The FMCS Experience," Labor Law Journal 27 (July 1976): 394.

27. Personal communication to the authors from Department of Research, Federal Mediation and Conciliation Service, September 26, 1978.

28. Office of Technical Services, Federal Mediation and Conciliation Service, letter to the investigators, February 15, 1977. The northeastern states including New York, New Jersey, Connecticut,

and Massachusetts accounted for approximately 50 percent of the 159 BOIs established by the beginning of 1978.

29. See Columbus Printing Pressmen and Assistants Union No. 252, 219 NLRB 54 (July 18, 1975). The NLRB has recently ruled that interest arbitration is not a mandatory subject for bargaining. Thus, in the Chicago situation, either of the parties could allow the clause to lapse and refuse even to discuss renewing it.

30. Contract Agreement between Twin City Hospitals and Minnesota Nurses Association, 1974-76, section 20, pp. 30-33.

31. Data supplied by the Division of Employee Relations and Training, American Hospital Association.

32. Ibid.

33. Ibid.

34. Hervey Juris et al., "Employee Discipline No Longer Management Prerogative Only," Hospitals, JAHA 51 (May 1, 1977): 71.

35. See, for example, Abraham Nash, "Labor Management Conflict in a Voluntary Hospital" (Ph.D. diss., New York University, 1972).

36. Report to the FMCS Health Care Industry Labor Management Advisory Committee, December 6, 1976.

37. See Ruth Howe Loevinger, "The Minnesota Story of Economic Security," American Journal of Nursing 51 (April 1951): 230.

38. Pointer, Unionization, p. 34.

39. See Norma K. Grand, "Nightingaleism, Employeeism, and Professional Collectivism," Nursing Forum 10 (1971): 290-91.

40. See Health Labor Relations Reports 1 (July 11, 1977): 5-6. That this point of view may be generally widespread was suggested by the results of a recent attitudinal survey of hospital administrators and union leaders. The authors of the study found that of 23 unions queried, 78 percent preferred "to settle their differences with management through binding arbitration rather than economic force." Nearly half the hospital managements responding to the survey were in agreement with this conclusion.

41. The classic statement of this phenomenon was made in Clark Kerr and Abraham Siegel, "The Interindustry Propensity to Strike—An International Comparison," in Industrial Conflict, ed. Arthur Kornhauser et al. (New York: McGraw-Hill, 1954), pp. 189-212.

42. See Ada Jacox, "Collective Action and Control of Practice by Professionals," Nursing Forum 10 (1971): 240-41. "In nursing, behavior 'unbecoming a lady' or contradictory to hospital policy has often been called unprofessional. To call something (sic) unprofessional has been a powerful means of controlling nurses, since their desire to be professional is so strong . . . to march, to

demonstrate, or to engage in similar activities have been inter-changeably called unprofessional, undignified, and unladylike."

43. See Norman Metzger and Dennis D. Pointer, Labor-Management Relations in the Health Services Industry (Washington, D.C.: Science and Health, 1972), p. 34.

7

THE UNION IMPACT ON
COMPENSATION IN HOSPITALS

In view of the spiraling costs of medical care, particularly among hospitals, policy makers have recently focused special attention on the hospital industry.[1] Blame for these developments frequently has been cast upon physicians, government bureaucracy, hospital administrators, and labor unions, among others. Yet while the rising costs of health care are all too apparent, the role of any or all of the participants mentioned above is not. The purpose of this chapter is to focus on the effect of one of these groups—labor unions—and attempt to identify its influence on the major component of hospital costs, the cost of labor. Since more than 50 percent of total hospital costs go to labor, the issue of union effects on compensation is particularly germane to this industry. If collective bargaining has raised wages to the same extent reported in other industries, the effect on health-care prices could be dramatic.[2] Noting the paucity of evidence on this issue, a recent study by the Wage and Price Council has called for "further research and analysis on the components of increases in medical costs and other relative contributions to inflation in the [hospital] sector. . . . [H]igher labor costs resulting from . . . collective bargaining . . . deserve special attention."[3]

While the literature is replete with studies of the union impact on manufacturing industries, little work has been done in the health field generally or the hospital industry in particular. In research on wage changes in the hospital industry, Martin Feldstein and Amy Taylor focused on the determinants of these changes in the 1960s but failed to explicitly consider the role of unionism.[4] Karen Davis finds little union effect on wages using cross-sectional data but has only indirect measures of union coverage.[5] David Salkever, using SMSA level data for the 1960s, concludes that "organization effects are greatest when [unions are present] but not widespread," suggesting the importance of potential threat effects.[6] Myron Fottler estimates wage effects of 4 to 8 percent for nonprofessionals using the same data source as Salkever, updated to 1972.[7] And finally, Charles Link and John Landen estimated union effects on the beginning salaries of registered nurses of 4.6 to 7.4 percent.[8]

This research is intended to expand on these earlier studies in several ways. First, it focuses on the industry subsequent to changes in the National Labor Relations Act and should, therefore, give a more accurate estimate of the current situation. Second, we expand our attention to the impact of unions on total compensation and not simply wages. This broader perspective is important because fringe benefits now make up more than 26 percent of total salary costs in the hospital industry.[9] As a result, to ignore the union effect on this substantial and growing aspect of compensation may result in a significant understatement of the union impact on total labor costs. The few studies that have considered the union effects on fringe benefits have tended to focus on manufacturing industries and are limited to an estimate of either the incidence of, or expenditures on, a particular fringe benefit (usually pensions).[10] In this study, the estimate will be analogous to the union wage differentials and include the value of all fringe benefits.

Finally, because of the unique data set, this research offers a means to partially measure the elusive effects of unionism on nonunion workers. These estimates can be important because, while it is not likely that the hospital industry will ever be organized to the same extent as the manufacturing sector, significant spillover and threat effects could spread union influence far beyond its own membership.

WAGES

Conceptual Framework

An analysis of the likely union effects on relative wages is typically framed in the context of the elasticity of demand for union labor. Despite a presumed inelastic demand for hospital services, the magnitude of these effects is somewhat uncertain. For example, nonprofessionals, whose jobs are essentially unskilled or semiskilled, are vulnerable to replacement in the event of a strike by either expanded efforts within the hospital or by hiring additional labor from the external labor market. In addition, while their presence is important to the smooth functioning of the hospital, their absence is not immediately life threatening and, therefore, as a group not as essential as more highly skilled labor.

Furthermore, because these workers make up a large part of the hospital labor force, the marginal costs of a union gain could be substantial. To the extent that administrators feel compelled to pass on some percentage of the union gain to maintain internal compensation structures, downward pressure on union gains would be created and the marginal cost of the bargain would exceed the increased compensation accruing just to unionized professionals.

The expectation for relatively modest union compensation gains is further underscored by the service workers' occupational structure. Particularly important are the poor opportunities for substantial on-the-job training and internal mobility as well as the large numbers of women and minorities in the service worker labor force. Lack of mobility within the hospital is a concern of unions representing these workers and may require a trade off of compensation demands if they are to be improved. While it could be argued that in the face of relatively poor opportunities for internal mobility unions would seek higher wages as compensation, the available evidence, though limited, suggests otherwise. Our interviews as well as other evidence suggest that unions representing service workers regard the "structuring" of the internal labor market as an important bargaining objective that may outweigh the concern for higher wages. [11] †

Similarly, to the extent that the large numbers of women are secondary wage earners and may lack the same tastes for unionism as primary wage earners, union leadership will not be able to take as hard a bargaining position as they would like—a position reinforced by the high turnover rates often associated with this group of workers. Moreover, both women and blacks could face fewer alternatives as a result of labor market discrimination and be more averse to the potential for job loss that might be associated with more aggressive bargaining tactics. [12]

Many of these same factors influence the position of professionals as well. For example, because general duty nurses are typically 30 to 40 percent of the hospital labor force, the marginal cost of a union wage gain is substantial. Even those professionals, such as pharmacists, who represent only a tiny portion of the work force may be constrained by a management policy of passing on union gains (at least in part) to nonunion workers.

Moreover, while professionals may possess more potential bargaining power (due to the essential nature of and lack of available

---

† As part of this research, interviews were conducted with a variety of hospital administrators, union officials, and interested third parties.

substitutes for their work) compared to service workers, the former may not have the same "tastes" for unionism or union tactics. Not only might professionals be less likely to join a union in the first place, but once organized they may be more reluctant to withhold their labor. It can be argued that these individuals have a greater identification with management, perceive themselves as "professionals" and thus above union activity, and, finally, have a closer relationship to the patient, making them more aware, both professionally and personally, of the effect of any strike.

Estimation Framework: Wage Model

Conventionally, the appropriate wage model is derived from the assumption that the average wage (W) is a weighted average of the competitive wage rate (W^c), the union effect on nonunion wages (R^n), and the union effect on union wage levels (M).[13] Expressing the variables in natural logarithms, we have

$$\ln \overline{W} = \ln W^c + \ln (1 + R^n) + U \ln (1 + M),\qquad(1)$$

where

$R^n = (W^n - W^c)/W^c$, where W^n = nonunion wages; U = measures of union coverage; and $M = (W^u - W^n)/W^n$, where W^u = average union wage.

If the model is put in terms of observables, then

$$\ln (W) = \sum_{n=1}^{k} a_n x_n + \lambda U = e,\qquad(2)$$

where $\sum_{n=1}^{k} a_n x_n$ is the sum of determinants of $\ln W^c$, U is the union coverage measure, e is a stochastic disturbance term, and λ is the effect of unionism on relative wages.[†] Customarily, the threat effect $(1 + R^n)$ is assumed to be included in e with the assumption that λ will not be biased. In this research, an effort will be made to measure explicitly the effect of unions on nonunion wages in union hospitals and reduce the likely bias in λ.

The following model will be used for estimation purposes:

$$\ln W = a_0 + a_1 U + a_2 (NU * UH) + a_3 Y + a_4 TO + a_5 SEX + a_6 RACE$$
$$+ a_7 SIZE + a_8 TEACH + a_9 POP + a_{10} GOVPER$$
$$+ a_{11} MONOP + e.\qquad(3)$$

[†]More accurately $\lambda = \ln(1+M)$, where [antilog (λ) - 1] equals M or the union/nonunion differential.

The reference categories for the dummy variables include,

The hypotheses are

$$a_1, a_2, a_3, a_7, a_8, a_9, a_{10} > 0; a_4, a_5, a_6, a_{11} < 0,$$

where W is the average occupational wage. Measures serving as independent variables include 1970 median county income (Y), average annual 1975 turnover rate for the occupation (TO), percent of the occupational labor force who are women (SEX) and minorities (RACE), number of beds in the hospital (SIZE), 1970 county population (POP), percent of third-party payer revenue derived from government sources (GOVPER), and a monopsomy measure defined as SIZE/total short-term beds in the county (MONOP). The remaining independent variables are coded as dummy variables and include the following: if the occupation is covered by a collective bargaining contract, U; if the occupation is a nonunion job in a union hospital, NU * UH; and if the hospital is an approved teaching hospital, TEACH. [†]

Two measures will be employed to determine the influence of unionism on wages. U, which will indicate if the occupation is covered by a collective bargaining agreement, is designed to pick up the direct union effects on the wages of its members. That this effect will be positive is the conventional wisdom. The real research interest involves the magnitude of this estimate.

Indicating a nonunion occupation in a union hospital, NU * UH represents indirect union effects on wages. Therefore, a_2 will reflect the relative wage differences between nonunion workers in union hospitals and their counterparts in a nonunion hospital. It is expected that a_2 will be positive, with the magnitude determined by both "threat" and "spillover" effects on nonunion labor. While it may not be particularly clear when a union gain is "threatening" and when it is "spilling over," it will be assumed that a threat effect implies hospitals have raised the wages of nonunion employees to prevent their unionization. Spillover effects, on the other hand, reflect a personnel policy change (that is, higher wages) designed to

---

[†]The reference categories for the dummy variables include, nonunion occupations, occupations in nonunion hospitals, and non-teaching hospitals. For the purposes of this analysis a hospital is considered a teaching hospital if it is a member of the Council of Teaching Hospitals of the Association of American Medical Colleges. Hospitals were considered union hospitals if on the survey questionnaire they answered "yes" to the question, "Are any of your employees currently covered by a union contract?"

retain a given structure and/or influence morale and feelings of equity among nonunion employees.

These two measures should pick up the bulk of the union influence on nonprofessional wage rates. However, they will not account for threat effects stemming from the external market. Because nonunion wages both in and out of union hospitals may be influenced, these effects are in part captured by NU * UH, though in all likelihood not completely so. Given our conversations with hospital administrators and the strong indication that nonunion hospitals attempt to "lead" the market, it is likely that both a_1 and a_2 are somewhat understated.

Control Variables

The hypotheses for the remaining independent variables were noted previously. At this point, we will simply provide a brief summary of the rationale for those hypotheses and reserve any further discussion for those results that might conflict with the expected effects.

Y serves as a proxy for different levels of demand for hospital services and, therefore, hospital labor. The direction of the effect is suggested by conventional economic theory where it is assumed, ceteris paribus, that higher income will result in a higher demand for hospital services. Moreover, Y will partially control for geographic differences in prevailing wages and cost of living.

TO can also be expected to influence wage levels. As others have noted, turnover represents a cost to employers, not only directly through recruitment and training outlay, but indirectly through the lost opportunity to reap the benefits of whatever firm-specific skills the worker may have possessed.[14] Employers will reduce wages where they are not able to capture these returns to firm-specific skills due to worker instability. In addition, turnover will lower the average wage rate of an occupational group by increasing the number of individuals at entry levels.

Furthermore, it is argued that teaching hospitals will not only seek out the most capable employee as a result of a greater concern for labor quality, but that more productive employees will want to work at such a hospital as either a source of human capital investment or simply professional pride. The result should be higher wages in these hospitals.

An attempt is also made to control demographic differences in the hospital labor force. Part of the typical human capital model of wage determination will include demographics such as sex and race. The expected lower average wages for these groups are hypothesized to be the result of (1) direct occupational discrimination and (2) differences in current productivity that are attributed in part to premarket discrimination.

SIZE should be positively related to wages if larger hospitals are able to generate more surplus through economies of scale and fund raising than their smaller counterparts. This in turn would allow these hospitals to pass on part of this surplus in the form of higher wages. Size can also influence wages if larger hospitals develop more professional personnel practices and in turn seek higher quality labor. Finally, it may be that organization size may serve as a negative, nonpecuniary aspect of work and, therefore, higher wages will be required to induce workers to enter the firm. In an interindustry study of plant size and wages, Stanley Masters made essentially these same arguments and found that plant size had at least as important an effect on wages as market structure.[15]

POP acts as a proxy for several potential positive effects on wages. First, it will pick up part of the differences in money wages not associated with the income measure, the assumption being that the cost of living is generally higher in urban areas. Second, it can be argued that urban areas offer more opportunities and, therefore, will attract a higher quality of labor. This would be particularly true for those who might be especially career-oriented and find greater opportunities for mobility and skill development in the city. Third, urban hospitals may have to pay a premium to offset the nonpecuniary disadvantages of city life and the added costs of commuting time. Finally, because POP also controls for the fact that population is likely to be associated with unionism and wages, it serves to reduce the bias (probably positive) in the union coefficient.

Wages and, in fact, all operating costs may also vary by the extent to which the hospital is reimbursed by third-party payers, particularly governmental sources. The argument tentatively would be that because hospitals are able to pass on wage increases to these governmental insurers and ultimately the consumer, hospital administrators would have less incentive to resist a wage increase. This hypothesis, however, is at best uncertain.

A measure of monopsony will be included because standard economic theory predicts that a monopsonist confronts an upward sloping supply curve, and will therefore pay less than the competitive market wage rate. However, given that monopsony, as measured in this study, will be greater in rural areas, the magnitude of the effect is uncertain. To the extent that these smaller rural hospitals offer a different or lower cost product and this characteristic is not completely controlled for by the other variables, a_{11} will be negatively biased and overstate the true effect.[16]

FRINGE BENEFITS

Conceptual Framework

While the union wage rate is the traditional focus of the union impact on labor costs, to ignore the union influence on fringe benefits would be to seriously understate the union effect on <u>total</u> compensation. Given that fringe benefits now represent nearly 37 percent of total compensation in many industries, the magnitude of this cost has become quite important. [17]

Despite the recent growth in these benefits, there is surprisingly little analytical attention given to them in the literature. Drawing upon the work of Gary Becker, Bevars Mabry concludes that where compensation is in the form of a deferred payment, worker stability should increase, a prospect particularly appealing to firms with high turnover costs due to the loss of firm-specific skills. [18] Similarly, fringe benefits are also "cheaper" than wages in that they do not increase with overtime and are not subject to payroll tax. Robert Rice notes that fringe benefits are more beneficial to workers as their rate of income taxation increases, because they are either nontaxable or received at a later point when a more favorable tax rate may be available. [19]

One of the most common strands throughout the literature in this area has been the focus on unionization as a likely determinant of fringe benefits. Rees comments, "There is some statistical evidence suggesting that the growth of fringe benefits has been particularly rapid in unionized employment."[20] He suggests that union leaders prefer such benefits as a bargaining objective, because they represent "symbolic" victories that if figured out in terms of wage gains would go unnoticed by their members. He also points out that employers may be more amenable to fringe benefit increases because of the savings in turnover costs.

Mabry argues that unions are more likely to seek and <u>win</u> higher fringe benefit levels because they are less likely to distort the compensation structure, often require bureaucratic oversight and serve as justification for union administration, and are less attractive to new (and possibly antiunion) workers. Moreover, if unions are able to educate their members to the advantages of fringe benefits, they can increase member acceptance of, if not demand for them. [21] Finally, in light of the relative lack of militancy on the part of the unions in the tristate area, they may choose to accept fringe benefits as a substitute for higher wage gains. †

---

† The management response to fringe benefit demands that would encourage such substitution is illustrated by one administrator

More recently, Richard Freeman has suggested that the effects of unions on fringe benefits can be analyzed in the context of the "exit-voice" paradigm. He argues that because fringe benefits require sizable "set up costs" and by their nature resemble public goods within the firm, individuals cannot really bargain effectively for them.[22] Therefore, the collective voice of the trade union is both a more appropriate and more effective method of communicating worker preferences for fringe benefits.

Empirical Evidence

As mentioned earlier, the few studies that have considered the union effects on fringe benefits have tended to focus on manufacturing industries and be limited in scope. Typical of these is the work by Rice, who used earnings, unionization, turnover costs, firm size, sex, and age as independent variables. Both earnings and firm size were found to have positive effects on supplemental benefits. Unionization, turnover costs, and the demographic variables were all insignificant. Due to the large "impact" of earnings (measured by contribution to explained variance) Rice concludes that the data are most consistent with the "tax treatment" hypothesis.[23]

William Bailey and Albert Schwenk use unionism, earnings, and establishment size as independent variables, all of which turn out to be positively related to expenditures on retirement and insurance plans.[24] They note that even when earnings are held constant, higher supplemental benefits are related to greater unionization and establishment size. Firm size probably reflects not only the ability to pay but also economies of scale in the provision of many fringe benefits. They did find, however, that it was easier to predict the incidence of such plans rather than the expenditures on them. Loren Solnick has recently improved on this work by considering expenditures on pensions and health insurance as the dependent variables of interest. Using establishment data, Solnick finds the average union effect to be an increase of 24 percent for pension expenditures and 46 percent for insurance expenditures, over a wide variety of industries.[25]

Estimation Framework: Fringe Benefit Model

Because literature devoted to the estimation of the determinants of fringe benefits is limited, there are no commonly accepted estima-

---

who admitted that only recently had he become aware of the true cost of "another day off."

tion models, though earnings, unionism, and firm size have been somewhat consistent in their relationship to fringe benefit levels. As a result, the following equation is offered, with its principal focus being an attempt to calculate unbiased estimates of the various sources of union effects on fringe benefits and not to provide a general model of supplementary benefits. The control variables in Equation (4) are included with that purpose in mind.

$$FB = d_0 + d_1 W + d_2 U + d_3 (NU * UH) + d_4 MU + d_5 SIZE$$

$$+ d_6 SEX + d_7 Y + d_8 MONOP + d_9 POP + t. \tag{4}$$

FB is the total value of supplemental benefits/total compensation for the occupation and is designed to include the value of all fringe benefits, including "time off" with pay. Independent variables include the average occupational wage rate ($\overline{W}$), number of bargaining units in the hospital (MU), number of beds in the hospital (SIZE), percentage of total occupational employment who are female (SEX), 1970 median county income (Y), a monopsony measure defined as SIZE/total short-term general care beds in the county (MONOP), and 1970 county population (POP). Additional variables that were scaled as "dummies" include the occupation covered by a collective bargaining agreement (U), and a nonunion occupation located in a union hospital (NU * UH).[†]

Given our previous discussions and review of the available research, the following hypotheses are suggested:

$$d_1, d_2, d_3, d_4, d_5, d_7, d_9 > 0; \ d_6 < 0; \ d_8 = ?$$

The potential threat effect (d_3) is expected to be positive as in the wage equation, although it may be of lesser magnitude if information about changes in fringe benefit levels is not as easily available as that for wage levels. In some instances, of course, such as "days off with pay," the presence of this benefit would be all too obvious.

MU indicates a multiunion hospital and is measured as the number of bargaining units in the jth hospital. The expectation is that as the number of unions in the hospital increases, so will the level of fractional bargaining. This, in turn, ought to result in intrahospital whipsawing and higher benefits. The influence of this

---

[†]Reference categories for the binary variables include nonunion occupations and nonunion occupations in nonunion hospitals.

variable should be particularly strong for fringe benefits, which, because they are not as easily communicated to nonunion workers as wage changes, would be easier for management to adjust given union pressure.

GOVPER, TEACH, and RACE are excluded from the fringe benefit model because there is little reason to believe these variables would influence the level of these benefits, independent of their effect on wages. Since wages are included in the model, these effects will simply be part of the overall wage effect on fringe benefits.

Control Variables

While Rice found the effects of demographic variables to be insignificant, we would expect SEX to influence the level of supplemental benefits. First, it can be argued that as in the area of wages, women may receive lower fringe benefits than men as a result of discriminatory employee practices. This would most likely take the form of job discrimination through which women have been denied access to positions with higher fringe benefit levels. A second reason for lower fringe benefits among women is that their work practices may differ from those of men. If women have expectations of shorter working careers, they will be less likely to be concerned about deferred benefits.

In general, income and population variables will serve as proxies for cost-of-living differences that could reflect higher fringe benefits in high income, urban areas. POP would also represent varying amounts of information about fringe benefits where it is expected that (1) urban areas are likely to serve as the vanguard for new and different fringe benefit demands, and (2), because of the complexity of some of the fringe benefit plans, information about them may be slow to reach rural areas, thus accentuating urban-rural differences. It is not clear what effect monopsony may have on benefit levels. It may be that monopsonists pay lower fringe benefits (as in the case of wages). On the other hand, monopsonists may want to restrict mobility and put more stress on firm-specific, on-the-job training. As a result, no hypothesis is made a priori.

The models will be stratified by occupational group since occupation can serve as a proxy for both employee tastes and employer perception of turnover costs. Moreover, it can be argued that the more highly skilled occupations (nurses, professionals, and technical workers) have greater tastes for stability and working conditions and, therefore, will seek higher fringe benefits—not only because they may value these benefits more highly than will service workers, but also because the effective return is higher due to greater job stability.

Finally, it is suggested by Rice that employers will attempt to use supplemental benefits as an incentive for job stability among groups for which turnover is more costly.[26] The implication is that more highly skilled groups will have greater costs associated with their turnover in terms of selection and training expenses as well as the loss of firm-specific skills that would have accrued to the employer. As a result, we would expect the union effects to be greater among the more highly skilled groups because the direct costs to management are in part offset, ceteris paribus.

DATA

The primary source of data, as pointed out previously, was a mailed questionnaire sent to all 563 general-care, short-term hospitals in Illinois, Wisconsin, and Minnesota. One hundred forty-four hospitals returned the questionnaire, yielding a sample that appears to be representative of the union activity found in the population. For example, 25 percent of the hospitals in the sample were unionized compared to 24 percent in the population. While the responding hospitals tended to be somewhat larger than those in the population generally, the ratio of union to nonunion hospital size was nearly identical (50.8 percent versus 50.4 percent) for the two groups.[27]

The 12 occupations were divided into five occupational groups. These include service workers (kitchen helpers, maids or porters, nurse's aides, switchboard operators, and ward clerks); technical workers (licensed practical nurses, medical technologists, X-ray technicians); professionals (physical therapists, staff pharmacists); nurses (general duty nurses); and craft workers (stationary engineers). (Descriptive statistics for selected variables in the wage and fringe benefit models are reported in Table 7.1.) Since 144 usable questionnaires were returned, the potential sample size for each occupational group would be 144 times the number of occupations in each group. In the case of service workers, for example, this would be 144 x 5 = 720.

Missing observations resulted in a somewhat smaller sample size. The principal reason for this problem was that certain hospitals, particularly smaller ones, did not employ people in the occupation in question. This most often occurred with ward clerks, stationary engineers, physical therapists, and pharmacists. Where employees existed but data were not reported, missing data for some variables were predicted with independent variables not in the regression model. For example, occupational turnover or fringe

TABLE 7.1

Descriptive Statistics for Selected Variables

Occupation/Variable	Mean	Standard Deviation
Service		
Wage	3.06	.60
Percent female	.8897	.199
Percent minority	.1185	.2386
Union membership	.200	.401 ⸜
(NU * UH)*	.081	.272
Turnover	.237	.1859
Fringe benefit level	.1709	.0751
Professional		
Wage	7.46	2.11
Percent female	.411	.389
Percent minority	.027	.111
Union membership	.066	.249
(NU * UH)	.245	.431
Turnover	.1597	.255
Fringe benefit level	.1703	.0781
Technical		
Wage	4.47	.901
Percent female	.830	.247
Percent minority	.075	.176
Union membership	.090	.2868
(NU * UH)	.167	.373
Turnover	.175	.169
Fringe benefit level	.1712	.0743
Nurses		
Wage	5.22	.675
Percent female	.976	.088
Percent minority	.049	.124
Union membership	.125	.332
(NU * UH)	.132	.340
Turnover	.2145	.1135
Fringe benefit level	.1700	.0725
Craft		
Wage	5.52	1.55
Percent female	.0349	.1700
Percent minority	.0137	.050
Union membership	.201	.403
(NU * UH)	.0825	.276
Turnover	.164	.173
Fringe benefit level	.1719	.0762
Hospital and labor market		
Beds (SIZE)	225.47	210.50
Income	9858.8	1940.7
Government percent reimbursement	.471	.141
Teaching hospitals	.097	.296
Union hospital	.264	.441
Population (in thousands)	1375.1	2234.2
Beds/total beds in county	.460	.779

*1 if occupation is nonunion but located in a union hospital, 0 otherwise.
Source: Compiled by the authors from mailed questionnaire.

benefit rates were predicted from hospitalwide rates that were also available from the questionnaire. The observation was dropped if data on wage rates or unionism were missing.

RESULTS

Wages

The results of the wage regressions for the five occupational groups are reported in Table 7.2. While the estimates range from +7 percent for professionals to -7 percent for technical workers, only the 6 percent estimate for service workers and the -7 percent for technical workers are statistically significant at conventional levels. [†]

The estimates are in part a reflection of several forces acting to reduce the wage effect among more skilled groups. First, the most recent and vigorous union activity has been among unions representing (or attempting to organize) service workers rather than professionals. Second, the large spillover effects (NU * UH) for service workers suggest that administrators must think twice about concessions to the wage demands of unionized skilled groups, because they are apparently passed on to service workers as well.

The negative union effects for technical workers are primarily due to the LPNs in this group. In the tristate area, their position in the occupational structure is somewhat tenuous, and some administrators have speculated that they will be replaced in the future by registered nurses who have graduated from two-year programs. As a result, LPNs may well be trading off employment security for wages in their negotiations. As might be expected, the LPN unions themselves are typically not very strong, and many of those interviewed (both unions and management) speculated that LPN unions may be absorbed by the RNs or service workers in the future. Taken together, these factors contribute to the observation of lower wages among unionized LPNs and technical workers.

Nonunion service, technical, and nursing personnel all experience positive (and statistically significant) wage effects from working in union hospitals. In each of these groups, the spillover effect exceeds the direct union member effect and tends to increase

---

[†]The "union effects" are calculated as the [antilog (a_1) -1]. Where a_1 is less than .10, the observed coefficient approximates, though slightly understates, this effect.

in magnitude as skill level declines. These effects range from 4.8 percent among nurses to 7.4 percent for service workers.

The source of these gains to nonunion workers appears to be primarily a spillover effect from other unionized groups within a hospital. It is likely that hospitals have sought to preserve their compensation structure in the face of union gains among some groups and, therefore, have passed these increases on to other occupations. However, the margin by which a_2 exceeds a might usefully be thought of as a threat effect to which hospitals have added a slight premium above the union spillover in order to buy off any tendencies toward unionism.

In general, the coefficients of the other variables were in the expected direction with some interesting exceptions. While the effects of turnover were mixed, their statistical insignificance and small magnitude suggest minimal costs of turnover in terms of lost returns to the hospitals of firm-specific skills. As expected, the effects of female employment ratio (SEX) were generally negative except for service workers. For this group, as well as the others, the coefficient often reflects poor control for individual job differences within each occupational class. For example, among service workers there was a higher percentage of women in the higher wage jobs, those of ward clerks and switchboard operators. †

Another surprising result is the negative effect that increasing government funding appears to have on wages. This may be due to the fact that hospitals receiving large quantities of government insured patients reflect the poverty areas they serve. Thus, we would expect (1) less skilled labor available; (2) lower ability to pay;

---

†Occupational dummies are not included in either the wages or the fringe benefit models because our interest is in estimating the total effect of the demographic variables on these dependent variables. With occupation in the model we only observe the effect of sex on wages, holding occupation constant. Yet the influence of sex on occupational level is probably a much larger part of the total sex wage differential. By excluding occupation we observe this combined effect.

Similarly, because occupational and sex distribution is so highly correlated with average wages in the five service occupations as well as occupational union coverage ($r = .75$ and $-.63$, respectively), SEX minimizes the possibility of bias in the union coefficient. Since low wage occupations (maids, porters, kitchen helpers, and so forth) are more highly unionized, the bias that does remain probably results in a slight understatement of the true union effect.

TABLE 7.2

Wage Model Regression Results

(Dependent variable: Natural logarithm for the average hourly money wage rate)

Independent Variables	Models				
	Service Workers	Technical	Nursing	Professionals	Craft
Constant	.6034[a]	1.4318[a]	1.332[a]	2.1406[a]	.8033[a]
	(.0517)	(.0859)	(.0946)	(.1654)	(.2533)
Union membership (U)	.0586[a]	-.0694[c]	.0319	.0728	-.00193
	(.0141)	(.0375)	(.0241)	(.0868)	(.0761)
(NU * UH)	.0723[a]	.0690[a]	.0463[c]	-.0331	-.0808
	(.01905)	(.0256)	(.0253)	(.0487)	(.1101)
Percent turnover (TO)	.0106	-.0577	.0768	-.1613[b]	-.0400
	(.0285)	(.05511)	(.0681)	(.0736)	(.1550)
Percent female in ith occupation (SEX)	.0453[c]	-.2263[a]	.0412	-.2713[a]	-.0162
	(.0260)	(.0361)	(.0773)	(.0489)	(.1673)
Percent minority (RACE)	.0101	.0657	.2140[a]	-.1506	.0020
	(.0251)	(.0578)	(.0658)	(.1762)	(.5648)

Governmental percent of third-party payments (GOVPER)	-.0961[a] (.0395)	-.1271[c] (.0709)	-.0467 (.0571)	-.1586 (.1501)	.2263 (.2303)
Income (Y)	.000038[a] (.0000037)	.000022[a] (.0000067)	.000021[a] (.0000055)	.0000096 (.000013)	.000069[a] (.000019)
Beds (SIZE)	.00021[a] (.000046)	.00031[a] (.000084)	.00020[a] (.000068)	-.000227 (.000158)	.00032 (.00024)
Teaching hospitals (TEACH)	-.04802[c] (.0293)	-.0741 (.0520)	-.0916[b] (.0426)	.0708 (.1021)	-.1210 (.1554)
Population (in thousands) (POP)	.000029[a] (.0000029)	-.000010[b] (.0000051)	.0000051 (.0000042)	.0000031 (.0000096)	.000010 (.000013)
Beds/total beds in county (MONOP)	.00253 (.00676)	.0081 (.0127)	-.01183 (.00963)	.01225 (.0225)	-.00424 (.0350)
N	487	317	107	153	86
$\bar{R}^2$	.6267	.3450	.6076	.2196	.2755

[a]Significant at .01 level.
[b]Significant at .05 level.
[c]Significant at .10 level.
Note: The standard error of the regression coefficient is reported in parentheses.
Source: Compiled by the authors from mailed questionnaire.

and (3) a different (lower cost) product offered. All three of these factors contribute to lower wages and are partially reflected by the government reimbursement variable. Similar results are reported elsewhere and suggest, without indicating a causal relationship, that many of the same characteristics that contribute to lower costs are also associated with greater amounts of government funding. [28] The problem is one of omitted variable bias.

The effects of hospital size, county income, and population were all in the expected direction. However, contrary to our hypothesis, teaching hospitals apparently pay 5 to 10 percent <u>lower</u> wages than nonteaching hospitals. The assumption was that the wage data reported by these hospitals would not include students and this may not have been the case. However, this explanation would apply only to the results for the nursing and technical fields. It may also be that because of the higher overall costs associated with running a teaching hospital, administrators in these hospitals may make an extra effort to cut costs wherever possible—in this case at the expense of labor.

And finally, as measured, monopsony is apparently an unimportant influence on wage rates. However, a good part of the reason for this lack of effect is due to the fact that the variable is highly correlated with hospital size, population, and income, which were also included in the model.

While it appears that unions have a small positive effect on hospital wages in these three states, we should note that the single equation model ignores the possible endogeneity of turnover and unionism. In fact, a more theoretically complete model would estimate the wage equation as follows:

$$W = f_1(U, TO, Z), \tag{5}$$

$$U = f_2(TO, W, X), \tag{6}$$

$$TO = f_3(U, W, K), \tag{7}$$

where W_i = natural logarithm of average wage rate in the ith occupation; $U_i = 1.0$ if ith occupation is unionized, 0.0 otherwise; TO_i = turnover rate in the ith occupation; and Z, X, and K are vectors of control variables. Results from a sample of service workers suggest that, in fact, the single equation estimates may overstate the true effects. An alternative estimation procedure using two-stage least squares yielded an estimated union effect less than one-eighth the size of the ordinary least squares coefficient. †

_____

†See Appendix for a complete discussion of this issue. While this more comprehensive estimation process indicates that the

Fringe Benefits

The regression results for separate occupational groups are reported in Table 7.3. They indicate, unlike the regression results for wages, that union members among all groups enjoy relatively greater fringe benefits than do nonunion members. In addition, for all but one group (nurses), the estimates exhibit relatively high statistical significance and suggest a union effect of from 2.5 to 5.8 percentage points. Given mean fringe benefit levels in the neighborhood of 17 percent, these union effects are on the order of 9 to 25 percent—obviously much larger than the union wage effects. †

The results also indicate that multiunion hospitals tend to pay lower fringe benefits than do nonunion or single union hospitals. This effect is apparently due to the fact that more than half of the multiunion hospitals are located in the Minneapolis area—an area where most of the union hospitals bargain on a multiemployer basis. This bargaining structure tends to reduce much of the internal whip-sawing that might prevail in single employer bargaining, and apparently provides sufficient countervailing power to minimize union gains. Moreover, faced with the prospect of several unionized groups within a hospital, an administrator will be pressured to use the fringe benefit gains of one group (union or nonunion) as the standard for another group. While this kind of equity consideration exists in any organization, an increase in the number of bargaining units should increase the prospect of such a spillover. Therefore, because the marginal cost of a fringe benefit increase for a given unit will go beyond the simple increase in their individual compensation bill, administrators may be more reluctant to grant the increase. ††

"direct" union effect is much smaller than reported in Table 7.2, at least for service workers the "total" effect is comparable, because union coverage tends to reduce turnover that in turn increases average wage rates.

†The union effects must be calculated by adding a_4 to either a_2 or a_3, because a unionized occupation or hospital implies a value of at least 1.00 for MU. MU is evaluated at 1.00 when calculating these effects because, for reasons discussed later, it seems to be the most representative estimate and is not distorted by the peculiar distribution of MU.

††The multiunion variable was not included in the results reported for the wage models, because its effect proved both statistically and practically insignificant. However, consistent with the fringe benefit results, when MU was included in the wage model, there was a slight upward movement in the union coefficients. The

TABLE 7.3

Fringe Benefit Model Regression Results
(Dependent variable: Fringe benefits/total compensation)

Independent Variables	Models				
	Service Workers	Technical	Nursing	Professionals	Craft
Constant	.0614[a] (.0237)	.0478[c] (.0294)	.0518 (.0837)	.0803[b] (.0393)	.0807[b] (.0403)
Wage (W)	.0071 (.0068)	.0071 (.0044)	.00056 (.0114)	-.0011 (.0026)	-.0042 (.0052)
Union member (U)	.0254[a] (.0101)	.0399[b] (.0171)	.0363 (.0339)	.0582[b] (.0307)	.0561[b] (.0275)
(NU * UH)	.0159 (.0124)	.0191 (.0126)	.0205 (.0216)	.0279 (.0177)	-.0061 (.0253)
Number of unions in hospital (MU)	-.0103[a] (.0034)	-.0119[a] (.0045)	-.0125 (.0095)	-.0160[a] (.0064)	-.0127 (.0086)
Monopsony (MONOP)	.0032 (.0039)	.0012 (.0051)	.0019 (.0084)	-.00076 (.00685)	.00095 (.0094)

Beds (SIZE)	.00099^a (.000017)	.00009^a (.00023)	.00011^a (.000039)	.000113^a (.000031)	.000091^b (.000043)
Percent female (SEX)	-.00038 (.0138)	.01865 (.0143)	.0482 (.0674)	.00144 (.01481)	-.0039 (.0376)
Income (Y)	.0000055^a (.0000018)	.0000044^b (.0000023)	.0000034 (.0000040)	.0000058^c (.0000034)	.0000078^c (.0000043)
Population (POP)	.0000054^a (.0000016)	.0000068^a (.0000018)	.0000073^b (.0000031)	.0000080^a (.0000025)	.0000081^a (.0000033)
N	619	388	136	196	109
$\bar{R}^2$	.234	.221	.187	.2476	.2614

[a]Significant at .01 level.
[b]Significant at .05 level.
[c]Significant at .10 level.

Note: The standard error of the regression coefficients is in parentheses.

Source: Compiled by the authors from mailed questionnaire.

These data also indicate that positive indirect union effects (threat and/or spillover) exist in all occupational groups except craft workers (see Table 7.4). The results suggest that nonunion members in union hospitals can expect up to 7 percent greater fringe benefit levels than their counterparts in nonunion hospitals. While the result for craft workers is negative, the coefficient does not even exceed its standard error, making any inferences uncertain. Similarly, while the estimates for the other groups are more stable, they are not significant by conventional standards. This is no doubt in part due to the high level of multicolinearity involved where intercorrelations typically range from .5 to .8.

TABLE 7.4

Union Impact on Fringe Benefits of Nonunion
Occupations in Union Hospitals
(in percentages)

Occupational Group	Threat–Spillover Effects
Service	3.0
Professional	7.0
Technical	4.3
Nurse	4.7
Craft	−10.0

Source: (Calculated from Table 7.3.)

Unlike the results for the wage equations, the indirect union effects are not as large as the direct union effects. Part of this difference may be explained by the fact that information about fringe benefits is not as readily available or understandable to nonunion workers, and, therefore, management may feel less pressure to pass on these union gains.[29]

As for the remaining variables in the model, although not all of the hypotheses were supported, there were no conflicts of any

---

decision was made to omit MU in the wage model because the slight bias that may have resulted was more than offset by the improved stability of the estimates.

consequence. The expected positive relationship between fringe benefits and wages was reported in only three of the five occupational groups, but in only two of these instances did the coefficients exceed the standard error. For those two groups (service and technical workers), a $1.00 increase in wages is associated with approximately a 4 percent increase in supplemental benefits.

A possible explanation for the observed relationship (or lack of it) between wage and other occupation-specific variables such as SEX, is that, at least as indicated in the questionnaire responses, it appears that there is little variation in fringe benefit levels within the hospitals. It is not clear whether this lack of variation is the true compensation policy of hospitals or merely an artifact resulting from the manner in which the questionnaires were filled out. In any event, most but not all of the variation is between hospitals and will be explained by hospital and environmental characteristics. †

Both the MONOP and SEX variables are insignificant in each sample. Notwithstanding the above caveat with respect to the female/male occupation employment ratio, it is interesting to note that the coefficient in the nurses' sample is nearly three times the magnitude of those in other samples. While we cannot accept the hypothesis that it is different from zero with much confidence, the relative size would suggest that in nursing, as might be expected because of the commitment required for training, women are more likely to be concerned about the benefits of job stability. In addition, part of the reason for the high standard error is the lack of variation in SEX where the standard deviation of .08 (for nurses) is not even 10 percent of the .97 mean.

Excepting the insignificance of median county income in the nurses and professional sample, hospital size, median county income, and county population all exhibit highly stable relationships with fringe benefit levels and are consistent with our hypothesis. As expected, large hospitals do offer greater fringe benefits and the rate is quite similar for all groups. For example, given a mean size of 235 beds, a one standard deviation change in size (approximately 200) would be associated with a 10 to 11 percent change in fringe benefits, on average.

The effect of living in a highly populated urban area was just as striking. The difference in benefit levels between Cook County (Chicago) and a rural county of 100,000 would be on the order of 19

---

†There must, of course, be some intrahospital variation given the results for the union member and nonunion member interaction variable since they too relate to occupation.

to 28.5 percent, depending on the occupational groups—an effect nearly twice that observed in the wage equation. It may be that, as in the internal market, information about fringe benefits is not as available as it is for wages, and, therefore, we are not as likely to find rural areas becoming aware of any changes.

Finally, median income, like population, serves as a proxy for cost-of-living differences and is positively associated with fringe benefit levels. A one standard deviation increase in median county income (nearly $2,000 from a mean of slightly less than $10,000) would indicate an increase in fringe benefits of 5.2 to 8.2 percent.

CONCLUSION: THE UNION EFFECT ON COMPENSATION

From the previous discussion, we can estimate the overall effect of unionism on total compensation. To do so, we must first consider the net effect on total compensation, which requires that we weigh the direct and indirect (NU * UH) union effects on wages and fringe benefits by (1) the percentage of each occupational group (service, nurses, and so forth) that is unionized (in a union hospital); (2) the relative size of that group in the hospital labor force; and (3) the size of the average occupational wage compared to the overall hospital average. We then get a 5.0 percent effect on wages and a 10.9 percent effect on fringe benefits. † Because fringe benefits are typically 20 percent of total compensation, these effects are then weighted by a four to one ratio resulting in a net effect of 6.1 percent on total compensation.

However, because our individual occupations do not include all of those in a typical hospital, we must consider the union effect on the remaining workers. We could attribute the average spillover effect (2.4 percent) to each group and then estimate the percentage

---

†The reader should keep in mind that the dependent variable (FB) is equivalent to fringe benefit expenditures/fringe benefit expenditures + wages (W). Therefore, the union effects reported here reflect the influence on this ratio and not simply the absolute level of fringe benefits. While this is the most common standard by which benefits are measured to determine the effect on "expenditures," one must incorporate the union effect on wages as well. For example, in the case of service workers, given a 9 percent union effect on FB and a 6 percent effect on W, the impact on fringe benefit expenditures is on the order of 16.7 percent.

of total manpower they constitute, assuming a rate of pay equal to the hospital average. Because we have included service workers and nurses, it is likely that up to 80 percent of the hospital labor force has been covered by the survey, resulting in an adjusted compensation effect of [.80 · .061 + .2 · .024] 5.35 percent.

If we assumed this omitted group was unaffected by unionism and that it consisted of up to 30 percent of the hospital staff, the overall union effect would still be [.7 · .061 + .3 · 0] 4.27 percent. While this figure may serve as a lower bound estimate, two points should be made. First, since our occupational groups (service, professional, and so forth) include all potential allied manpower staff, we might assume a distribution of those not included in the study among those groups that is relatively equal to the distribution in the sample, in which case the original 6.1 percent estimate would be appropriate. Secondly, because the absolute magnitude in the difference of these estimates is so small (that is, 1.73 percent), there is little practical consequence. For purposes of discussion, therefore, we will use the 5.35 percent figure calculated in the second example.

While the magnitude of the compensation effect is important, we can by no means conclude that unions are much of a factor in wage inflation for hospitals in the tristate area. In general, the unions in each of the states are characterized by a lack of militancy that partially explains the size of the estimates compared to those in manufacturing. We cannot say that this same relationship will necessarily hold for labor markets in which more militant unions operate or that it will continue in the future when the effects of the 1974 amendments to the NLRA can more accurately be assessed.

While this chapter has provided some evidence of the union impact on compensation, a later chapter will consider how this impact and other union effects are translated into changes in hospital-operating costs. The intention is to paint a total picture of the union relationship to hospital costs by identifying not only the sources of any union effects, but also the magnitudes.

NOTES

1. Martin Feldstein and Amy K. Taylor, The Rapid Rise of Hospital Costs (Washington, D.C.: Council on Wage and Price Stability, 1977), p. 7. During the 1966-76 period, hospital charges rose 264 percent compared to an increase of 76 percent in the overall Consumer Price Index and show little sign of abating.

2. For a review of this literature see Geoege Johnson, "Economic Analysis of Trade Unions," American Economic Review 65 (May 1975): 23-28.

3. Bureau of National Affairs, "The Problem of Rising Health Care Costs," Daily Labor Report, no. 81 (August 26, 1976), pp. X1 to X15.

4. See Martin Feldstein, Rising Cost of Hospital Care (Washington, D.C.: Information Resources Press, 1971) and Amy K. Taylor, "The Demand for Labor in Non-Profit Institutions: Studies of the Hospital Industry" (Ph.D. diss., Harvard University, 1974). Feldstein attributes the wage increases primarily to "philanthropic" behavior on the part of hospitals. Taylor claims to explain 80 to 85 percent of the wage change during the 1958-67 period. However, by omitting unionization from her model, the positive effects of several included variables may be biased.

5. Karen Davis, "Theories of Hospital Inflation," Journal of Human Resources 8 (Spring 1973): 67-75. Because no direct union measures were available, Davis used a dummy variable indicating whether or not the state had favorable labor laws. The percent of nonagricultural employment unionized was also included. Both are poor measures of hospital union membership, and it is not surprising that her findings were not significant.

6. David S. Salkever, "Hospital Wage Inflation: Demand Pull or Cost Push?," Quarterly Review of Economics and Business 15 (Autumn 1975): 41.

7. Myron D. Fottler, "The Union Impact on Hospital Wages," Industrial and Labor Relations Review 30 (April 1977): 342-56.

8. Charles Link and John Landen, "Monopsony and Union Power in the Market for Nurses," Southern Economic Journal 41 (April 1975): 649-59. These percentage effects were calculated from the reported data.

9. Bureau of National Affairs, Daily Labor Report, no. 243 (December 18, 1978), pp. 3-4, table 3.

10. These are Robert Rice, "Skill, Earnings and the Growth of Wage Supplements," American Economic Review 56 (May 1966): 583-94; William Bailey and Albert Schwenk, "Employee Expenditures for Private Retirement and Insurance Plans," Monthly Labor Review 95 (July 1972): 15-19; Bevars Mabry, "The Economics of Fringe Benefits," Industrial Relations 12 (February 1973): 95-106; Frank Stafford, "Concentration and Labor Earnings: A Comment," American Economic Review 58 (March 1968): 174-81; Duane Leigh, "Unions and Black-White Differences in the Wages and Fringe Benefits of Middle-Aged Men" (Paper prepared for Secretary of Labor's Invitation Conference on the Longitudinal Surveys of the Pre-Retirement Years, Washington, D.C., August 1976); and Loren Solnick, "Unionism and Fringe Benefit Expenditures," Industrial Relations 17 (February 1978): 102-7.

11. For a discussion of union interest in "structuring" the internal labor market, see Jack Barbash, "The Emergence of Union Low-Wage Unionism," in Proceedings of the Twenty-Sixth Annual Winter Meeting of the Industrial Relations Research Association, ed. Gerald G. Somers, pp. 275-83. Madison: Industrial Relations Association, 1973.

12. Fottler, "Union Impact," pp. 343-44, argues that union-ized nonprofessionals, in fact, face an inelastic demand for labor. Moreover, he suggests that since minorities and women have re-cently made relatively greater union gains in manufacturing indus-tries, the wide representation of these groups among hospital non-professionals implies potentially large union wage effects. However, it is more likely that those gains have stemmed from flat rate settle-ments and the concentration of these groups in low wage jobs (re-sulting in high percentage effects) rather than any identifiable in-crease in their bargaining power.

13. This study employs the widely accepted estimation pro-cedure outlined first in H. Gregg Lewis, Unionism and Relative Wages in the United States (Chicago: University of Chicago Press, 1963) and later in Orley Ashenfelter, "Racial Discrimination and Trade Unionism," Journal of Political Economy 80 (May/June 1972): 435-64.

14. See, for example: George Johnson, "Economic Analysis of Trade Unions," American Economic Review 65 (May 1975): 23-28; Walter Oi, "Labor as a Quasi-Fixed Factor," Journal of Political Economy 70 (December 1962): 538-55; J. H. Pencavel, "Wages, Specific Training, and Labor Turnover in U.S. Manufacturing In-dustries," International Economic Review 13 (February 1973): 53-64; and Lyman Porter and Richard Steers, "Organization, Work and Personal Factors in Employee Turnover and Absenteeism," Psycho-logical Bulletin 80 (August 1973): 151-76.

15. Stanley Masters, "Wages and Plant Size: An Interindustry Analysis," Review of Economics and Statistics 51 (August 1969): 341-45.

16. It might also be argued that public versus private owner-ship would influence our results if ownership were correlated with both wages and unionism. For example, at the SMSA level, public ownership is positively correlated with wages and unionism; see Fottler, "Union Impact," p. 349. However, in this sample, the probability of public ownership is highly correlated with geographic location as the vast majority of counties in the three states have only one short-term general-care facility that is publicly owned. There-fore, both POP and MONOP would be highly correlated with the like-lihood of public ownership and minimize any potential bias in the union estimates. While the expectation is that any bias is quite

small, unfortunately it is not a testable assertion because the ownership data are not retrievable.

17. U.S. Chamber of Commerce, "Employee Benefits, 1977," reported in Bureau of National Affairs, Daily Labor Report, no. 243 (December 18, 1978), pp. 3-4. Note that while the Chamber of Commerce averages are calculated as fringe benefits/salary, our measure is fringe benefits/total compensation.

18. See Gary S. Becker, Human Capital: A Theoretical and Empirical Analysis with Special Reference to Education (New York: National Bureau of Economic Research, 1964); and Mabry, "Fringe Benefits." According to Becker, p. 19, this would be particularly true of monopsonists.

19. Rice, "Growth of Wage Supplements," pp. 584-90.

20. Albert Rees, The Economics of Trade Unions (Chicago: University of Chicago Press, 1963), p. 66.

21. Mabry, "Fringe Benefits," pp. 97-98.

22. R. B. Freeman, "Individual Mobility and Union Voice in the Labor Market," American Economic Review 65 (May 1975): 364-66.

23. Rice, "Growth of Wage Supplements," p. 588.

24. Bailey and Schwenk, "Employee Expenditures," p. 161.

25. Solnick, "Unionism and Fringe Benefit Expenditures," p. 104.

26. Rice, "Growth of Wage Supplements," pp. 583-85.

27. Nonresponse bias is an issue in surveys; however, the fact that some variables may be distributed differently in the sample than in the population does not necessarily bias the estimates on those variables in a regression model. That is, we can get unbiased estimates of the union effect on wages even if the variables are not distributed identically to the population. See Arthur Goldberger, "Selection Bias in Evaluating Treatment Effects: Some Formal Illustrations" (Discussion Paper #123-72, University of Wisconsin at Madison: Institute for Research on Poverty, 1972), p. 20. "The same linear function holds over the entire range of (X) and will be observed no matter what subrange of (X) we choose to observe. . . . (Nothing in the usual regression model requires that the distribution of the explanatory variable be representative of its distribution over the entire population.)" If the distribution of the dependent variable were truncated, the estimates could be biased. Such truncation, however, does not seem to be a problem given the range of hospitals in the sample.

Unfortunately, while these descriptive measures appear representative, we have no way of determining if there are significant differences in the conditional relationships for the response and nonresponse group. This, of course, would remain a problem had the response rate been even 60 or 70 percent.

28. Similar results were reported in David S. Salkever, "A Micro-Economic Study of Hospital Cost Inflation," Journal of Political Economy 80 (November/December 1972): 1158.

29. There are two conflicting forces operating to affect the standard errors of the regression coefficients in the fringe benefit model. The most important influence serves to reduce the standard errors below their true values. Because we have essentially a clustered sample (that is, each hospital questionnaire provides data on five separate service occupations), the observations are not totally independent. The wage model is also affected by this last influence, though to a lesser extent because of lower intracluster correlations. For a discussion of how this can result in inflated t-statistics, see Leslie Kish, "Confidence Intervals for Clustered Samples," American Sociological Review 22 (April 1957): 154-65. The potential effect is to reduce the coefficients to marginal statistical significance. A partially offsetting influence in the fringe benefit models is that, because a number of fringe benefit levels are predicted from the hospital average, measurement error is introduced that serves to inflate the standard error of the regression coefficients.

8

THE IMPACT OF
COLLECTIVE BARGAINING ON
HOSPITAL MANPOWER POLICIES

The cost of health-care manpower is a function of the productivity of hospital employees as well as the amount of compensation paid to them. A dominant fear among hospital administrators is that collective bargaining will severely curtail a hospital's ability to hire, promote, assign, reward, or discipline employees in what the administrators believe is the most efficient and rational manner. This issue, of course, is not restricted to the health-care industry but has existed historically in nearly all unionized sectors of the economy. Neil Chamberlain and Donald Cullen suggest that management rights have been the most fundamental issue in collective bargaining "since the first union served its demands upon an employer used to deciding for himself what the employment conditions should be in his own shop."[1]

The argument between labor and management results in a clash between management's right to run its business efficiently and profitably and the need for workers to have a voice in decisions affecting their jobs.[2] This need may be a result of general social values that encourage industrial democracy through workers' participation in management or be simply associated with job and income security, due process on the shop floor, or equitable treatment from supervisors.

Concrete expressions of this aspect of collective bargaining conflict are manifested first in the negotiation of management rights clauses in contracts and then through the establishment of grievance procedures and contractual constraints over such issues as subcontracting, crew size controls, distribution of overtime, use of seniority in personnel decisions, and exclusion of supervisors from performing work in the bargaining unit, to enumerate just a few of the possibilities.

112

Work rules that limit management's discretion may be viewed as "social justice" by workers and "featherbedding" by employers. As such, the struggle over management rights may be as much philosophic as economic—that is, involve matters of principle—and, therefore, be bitterly disputed by the parties.

In an industry such as the hospital, where unionization is only now emerging, hierarchical relationships have stressed loyalty and obedience to management, and employees have often worked under conditions of low pay and minimal job security. The ingredients are present, therefore, for a major confrontation over management's right to manage without interference.

Finally, it should be noted that government labor policy also contributes both to the origin of collective bargaining disputes over an employer's manpower policy as well as to their resolution. For example, it was pointed out in Chapter 5 that Congress specifically instructed the NLRB in 1974 to avoid the fragmentation of bargaining units in hospital work forces. To do otherwise would create a potential for jurisdictional disputes between unions, rigidity in work assignments and transfers, union "leapfrogging" in bargaining settlements, imbalances in internal wage structures, and, perhaps most importantly, discontinuity in patient care.

Federal labor policy also, however, has an impact through the duty-to-bargain sections of the Taft-Hartley law that prescribe the procedures for negotiations and the subjects that must be discussed. Thus, the parties, regardless of their wishes, must bargain "in good faith" over such subjects as job evaluation, discipline, subcontracting, and anything that generally can be placed under the rubric of "wages, hours, and other terms and conditions of employment." While it is not necessary to make concessions, it is an unfair labor practice to refuse to discuss prescribed topics. Management may find itself in the uncomfortable position of negotiating what rights or prerogatives it will continue to exercise unilaterally. If its bargaining power is weak vis-a-vis the union, these rights may be quite limited. †

---

†In a recent settlement between Los Angeles County Hospital and the Joint Council of Interns and Residents representing 1,300 housestaff, the words "management responsibilities" were added to "management rights" in the contract. Conflict over the clause "had been central to a stalemate in the negotiation of the new collective bargaining agreement."

MANAGEMENT RIGHTS IN HOSPITALS

Although management rights are a very significant matter for both labor and management in hospitals, there is only limited consensus among administrators on how to handle the issue.[3] For example, only 60 percent of hospital union contracts in the tristate area contain management rights clauses, in contrast to 75 percent of hospital contracts generally and 69 percent in all U.S. industry. The lack of agreement has been attributed to a state of uncertainty among managers themselves.

> Much of modern and progressively developing management practices involve democratic management—group problem solving—which particularly lends itself to hospitals, where highly skilled and trained professionals not only have the preeminent knowledge and skills to make these kinds of decisions but also will be encouraged to perform better if they participate in that kind of decision making. Perhaps the traditional standards of management rights need to be re-examined in the light of the health industry. . . .[4]

However, for many hospital managers whose position is not uncertain, intrusion of unions into management rights, particularly those relating to decisions about patient care, will be achieved only on the basis of strikes and job action. Existing management prerogatives will not be forgone voluntarily.

PATIENT CARE ISSUES IN COLLECTIVE BARGAINING

A review of the major job actions or strikes of professional health-care employees in recent years suggests that working conditions directly related to patient care have been at the base of disputes more often than have economic issues. For example, interns and residents struck Cook County Hospital in October and November 1975 over such issues as laboratory improvement guarantees, an end to out-of-title work, the training of nurses and paramedics to set up intravenous systems, and the creation of a health-care advisory committee equally divided between doctors and the hospital governing commission. Prior to the strike, the housestaff had presented more than 100 patient-care demands to an administration who argued that patient-care demands should not be subject to collective bargaining.[5]

In another case involving interns and residents, a major element in a settlement at the Los Angeles County health-care facilities was a stipulation that the county allocate $1 million to establish a patient-care fund to buy emergency medical supplies and to reactivate 11 intensive care unit beds that had been closed because of lack of nurses.[6] While shorter hours and salary increases also figured prominently in housestaff disputes in New York,[7] as well as Chicago and Los Angeles, demands concerning working conditions have generally been predicated on improving the quality of patient care.

Nurses also have been very much involved in disputes over patient-care related issues. Strikes and job actions have occurred in St. Louis, Chicago, San Francisco, and Seattle as well as in the smaller cities of Ames, Iowa, Willimantic, Connecticut, and Columbus, North Carolina, among others. Invariably, the bargaining demands have focused on staffing in addition to scheduling hours, shifts, weekends, and so-called out-of-title work.[8]

One of the longest and most bitter strikes of registered nurses was in Youngstown, Ohio early in 1975. Approximately 450 RNs stayed off the job for 53 days in a dispute with the Youngstown Hospital over the demand that the American Nurse's Association Code for Nurses be made a part of the new contract.[9] Specifically, the two sections of the Code under contention were:

> Provision 3—The nurse maintains individual competence in nursing practice, recognizing and accepting responsibility for individual actions and judgements.
> Provision 5—The nurse uses individual competence as a criterion in accepting delegated responsibilities and assigning nursing activities to others.

The nurses were unsuccessful in having the Code placed in the contract, although the hospital did agree to consider it as a factor in disputes arising from the refusal of nurses to accept specialized duty because of lack of training.[10]

The Youngstown strike was an example of a dispute over out-of-title work, an issue that has arisen not only with RNs but with housestaff as well. Efforts have been made through collective bargaining to limit such assignments as clerical tasks, drawing blood, setting up intravenous systems, and duties for which employees and staff professionals are ill trained or inexperienced.

Staffing issues have also been a source of contention between hospitals and their professional employees. In the opinion of one official of a nurses association, "Staffing is the major concern of most registered nurses."[11] Nurses point to Standard I of the Joint

Commission on Accreditation of Hospitals (JCAH) which states, "There shall also be sufficient number of duly licensed registered nurses on duty at all times to plan, define, supervise, and evaluate nursing care, as well as give patients the nursing care that requires the judgement and specialized skills of the registered nurse."[12] A level deemed sufficient by the administration, however, may be labeled as gross understaffing by the nurses. Since the JCAH standards are left to the hospital to implement, they can become an issue in bargaining.

Staffing issues have surfaced in hospital labor-management disputes not only regarding the employees involved in the negotiations but also in demands made concerning workers outside the bargaining unit in question. For example, housestaffs at times have sought increased employment of aides, LPNs, and RNs as a means of reducing the burdens and nonrelevant duties of interns and residents.

The cost and managerial implications of staffing and out-of-title bargaining demands are such that it is not surprising that hospital administrators have been adamant in their refusal even to discuss such issues, much less accept contractual limitations on what they consider their responsibilities. Their position is summarized in the following statement of the Executive Committee of the American Hospital Association:

> The staffing of a hospital must be an objective process and should not be controlled by a group with special interests. . . . Nurses as an organized group are not legally responsible for patient care. Only management has the responsibility to determine the number of employees, their qualifications, and their assignments within the institution so as to be consistent with the best patient care and the most effective utilization of personnel.[13]

Finally, it should be noted that procedures by which employees could participate in decision making also have been placed on bargaining tables. Interns and residents have demanded health-care advisory committees, and registered nurses have sought to acquire a voice in decision making through a variety of committee structures carrying such labels as professional staffing, professional performance, or joint study, to name a few. These efforts have been countered by the arguments of hospital management that such demands are neither bargainable nor related to patient care. At best, say the hospitals, these are merely "examples of an attempt by unions to mask economic demands in the form of patient care and quality of care issues."[14] At worst, so it is alleged, employee unions or associations are moving toward taking over complete control of the hospital.

In view of the importance attached to patient-care concerns by professional employees across the United States, it is surprising that these issues have not been a focal point for collective bargaining in the unionized private hospitals in Minnesota, Wisconsin, and Illinois. For example, only 30 percent of the 126 hospital contracts available to the investigators provided for sharing decision making through such devices as joint study committees. This figure is far below the 52 percent for all hospital contracts estimated from the Juris data. Moreover, in only 3 percent of sample contracts in the tristate area providing for joint study were the committees' recommendations binding.

Although comparable data are not available for Illinois, Wisconsin, and Minnesota, Juris's analysis of all U.S. hospital contracts suggests that where joint study committees are found, they are used most frequently by professional workers (73 percent) and least by nonprofessionals (16 percent). For technical employees, the comparable figure for use of joint study committees is 52 percent.[15] His findings thus provide mixed support for the argument raised by some management spokesmen that once professionals obtain the right to participate in management processes, "other unions within the organization would have every right to exert the same pressure and ultimately, through precedent, win their point."[16]

A related, and presumably more restricted, mechanism for joint participation is the labor-management safety committee. Although labor-management safety committees appear in nearly 40 percent of labor agreements throughout the United States, such committees are not frequently used in the hospital industry generally (13 percent) or in the hospitals of the tristate area (9 percent).

Although provisions for joint participation appear to be rare in hospital contracts, it is conceivable that they may nevertheless constitute a source of bargaining conflict. Pursuing this premise, examination of both strikes and bargaining controversy reveals little evidence for Illinois, Wisconsin, or Minnesota that either the process of decision making or the decisions themselves (as they involve staffing, out-of-title work, or related subjects) have been a major issue between the parties.

The exception to this generalization is the Cook County hospital complex of Chicago in which separate strikes by both nurses and housestaff have revolved around patient-care considerations. Cook County is a public hospital with very special problems. The conflict in this particular hospital does not seem to have had repercussions on other hospitals, private or public, in the three states.

Several factors seem to be at work in holding down the amount of labor-management conflict over patient-care decisions. First, professional and technical employees in Illinois and Wisconsin are generally not involved in collective bargaining in private sector hospitals. As the Juris data show, it is this segment of the hospital work force that is most interested in patient care and its implications for employment and working conditions.

Second, although Minnesota has a high proportion of hospital professionals organized, the climate for labor relations in recent years seems to be characterized by relatively good feelings between the parties. The hostility and militance so much in evidence in other areas is largely absent from the industrial relations systems of Minnesota hospitals.

A third factor contributing to the characteristic low profile given patient-care issues in the three states is the bargaining posture assumed by hospital managements. Where possible, they may offer economic benefits as a trade off for patient-care demands. If these demands cannot be bought off, then the hospital representatives may take a hard line. The only way management will concede is when forced to do so. Thus, the employees must be prepared to strike the hospital over such issues as staffing, out-of-title work, or joint study committees—a prospect not appealing in most circumstances. Speculation about whether this situation is likely to change in the future will be reserved for later in the chapter.

WORK RULES, JOB SECURITY, AND DUE PROCESS

The nonprofessional hospital worker often has little direct contact with patients. For those employees working in housekeeping, kitchen, laundry, or related activities, tasks assigned, supervision received, and hourly wage paid may differ little from unskilled or secondary labor market jobs in other service industries. Thus, participation in management patient-care decisions may have little value in collective bargaining compared to basic economic gains or provisions in a collective contract insuring job security and fair treatment. Hence, strong efforts may be made to limit management's discretion in decisions over layoffs, recall, promotions, and transfer, as well as to reduce the possibility that work can be removed from the bargaining unit. In addition, through the grievance procedure, a system of due process may be established to provide stringent guidelines for handling cases of discipline and discharge. Management's opposition to contractual constraints of this kind in its manpower activities may be less philosophic than administrative. The reward or retention of inadequate employees may be not only inefficient from the hospital's standpoint, but unsafe as well.

Probationary Status

One point at which the question of retention of unsatisfactory employees ordinarily is handled is during the probationary period. The longer the period, the more flexibility enjoyed by management but, conversely, the less job security possessed by the workers. Analysis of the hospital labor contracts available to us indicates that hospitals in the three states generally require long periods of probation; nearly half of the contracts specified between 60 and 90 days, and only 3 percent permitted 30 days or less.

Work Rules

Hospital labor contracts in the tristate area also appear to lack the controls over work rules often present in industrial-labor management agreements. As Table 8.1 indicates, the hospitals are free from constraints on subcontracting, can use supervisors to perform work in the bargaining unit, and can assign whatever numbers of individuals deemed appropriate to a task or machine. So-called crew size restrictions, to the extent they exist, are usually applied only to powerhouse employees.

Slightly more prevalent are contract clauses providing equal distribution of overtime, guarantees of hours and/or pay, and standby pay. Only half the contracts stipulated paid rest periods, and 45 percent of the hospitals had no contractual obligations to post jobs.

Instances of joint handling of issues such as safety and job evaluation are rare. Only 7 percent of the contracts permitted joint determination of wages by job evaluation, and an even smaller number accepted a similar procedure for job content.

Seniority in Employment Decisions

A controversial manpower question is the use of service or seniority to govern promotions. In its survey of union-management contracts, the Bureau of National Affairs reports that 69 percent provide that seniority will be a consideration in promotion decisions.[17] Juris indicates that the equivalent figure for all hospitals is 66 percent. However, as the determining factor in the promotion of hospital employees, seniority appears in 17 percent of the contracts in contrast to 38 percent of all labor agreements in industry.[18]

TABLE 8.1

Manpower Subjects Covered by Hospital Contracts
in the Tristate Area, 1976
(N = 126)

Issue	Percent of Contracts Mentioning
Subcontracting restriction	1.0
Crew size control	7.0
Supervisor performing work in bargaining unit	0.0
Provisions for job posting	55.0
Joint labor-management safety committees	9.0
Joint determination of wages by job evaluation	7.0
Joint determination of job content by job evaluation	4.0
Paid rest periods	51.0
Standby pay	45.0
Equalization of overtime	29.0
Guarantees of hours and/or pay	23.0
Superseniority	*

*Less than 1 percent.
Source: Compiled by the authors.

Seniority is also a factor in decisions concerning layoff, recall, and transfer, but, as the Juris data suggest, it apparently is used less often by hospitals than by industry generally (see Table 8.2).

Inspection of the seniority provisions of hospital labor contracts in Illinois, Wisconsin, and Minnesota reveals similarities as well as important differences with both other industries and the hospital industry elsewhere. In nonprofessional contracts, length of service is usually a secondary factor in promotions, layoffs, and recall; a common approach is to resort to seniority only where "ability and fitness" are equal among candidates. How much leeway permitted management is indicated by the following clause from a Wisconsin nonprofessional employee contract: "Promotions, transfers, and reductions of work force shall be based on the abilities, aptitudes, and work records of employees as determined by the hospital. Where these qualifications are equal, seniority shall become the determining factor." For the most part, no mention is made of seniority in the contracts of hospital professional workers. An exception is the case of the unionized radiologic technologists in Minnesota, whose contracts specify that straight seniority be used in cases of layoffs.

TABLE 8.2

Seniority as a Factor in Layoff, Recall, and Transfer in
Hospitals and All Industries, 1976
(in percentage of contracts)

	Hospitals	All Industries
Recall	66.0	75.0
Layoff	75.0	85.0
Transfer	44.0	48.0

Source: Hervey A. Juris, "Labor Agreements in the Hospital Industry: A Study of Collective Bargaining Outputs," in Proceedings of the 1977 Annual Spring Meeting of the Industrial Relations Research Association (Madison: Industrial Relations Research Association, 1977), p. 508.

It is customary in union-management agreements to provide union officials with superseniority, a position at the top of a seniority roster, to ensure that in the event of reductions in staff, union contractual obligations such as grievance handling can continue. Obviously, the greater the number of individuals protected from layoff, the more difficult it becomes to reduce labor costs as well as to insure that key jobs are adequately filled.

Superseniority is found in nearly 40 percent of the labor agreements in all unionized industries, but in only 11 percent of the contracts in the hospital industry generally. Of the 126 contracts in our tristate hospital sample, only one provided for superseniority.

Education and Training

A final issue having direct impact on a hospital's labor cost, and one that should be an important concern to all categories of employees, is the extent to which a contract requires the employer either to cover the cost of outside training for employees or to provide the training "in-house." On the one hand, professionals need to keep up with often rapid and significant changes in their practice. Nonprofessional employees, on the other hand, are frequently holders of low paying, dead-end jobs from which they can escape only by increasing their education and training. We would expect that unions and professional associations alike would place high priority on obtaining significant concessions in this area from hospital administrators.

In our examination of tristate hospital labor contracts, we were surprised to find this benefit mentioned only rarely; nor did there appear to be much effort to achieve it. More than 75 percent of the contracts had no provision for training either on a general basis or specifically for promotion. In those that had such provisions, the hospitals agreed to pay outside tuition in 33 percent of the cases and provided some type of in-house training in 20 percent. Two-thirds of the sample contracts even lacked a provision that would permit employees to take unpaid leaves of absence for educational purposes.

Discipline and Discharge

The drive for equitable treatment in the workplace may be directed not only at the dispensation of rewards but also to the meting out of discipline. Penalties must not be arbitrary in conception nor capricious in application. Mechanisms of challenge and appeal must be available and efficient.

The grievance procedure of a contract may be simultaneously a device for ensuring social justice and for vetoing or blocking managerial decisions. Thus, contractual provisions regulating the procedures and application of discipline and discharge in the hospital have important manpower implications for both parties.

In our sample of 126 contracts in the tristate area, 28 percent specified explicit procedures for notification of discharge; the procedure usually included notifying the union as well, although, at times, after the fact. This figure compares with 31 percent for hospital contracts generally, and 59 percent for all U.S. industries.[19] In the case of discipline short of discharge, only 11 percent of the contracts expressly provided that the employees or the union be informed of the nature of the rule infraction and the action taken. The comparable figures for all hospitals and all industry are both about 21 percent.

A second disciplinary procedural issue is whether records of disciplinary action should be removed after specified periods of time. While Juris found about 10 percent of all hospital contracts made provision for removal from employee records of instances of disciplinary action, in the tristate sample the proportion of hospital contracts addressing the issue was even smaller—about 3 percent.

Beyond the procedures established in labor agreements for handling discipline, it is also important to know whether the causes for discipline or discharge are also specified in the contract. Lack of such specification would, of course, provide hospital administrators with great flexibility in managing employees. Table 8.3 presents a list of potential causes for discharge by frequency with which they are mentioned in our sample of contracts. It should be noted that 68 percent of the agreements listed no specific cause; they either contained no provisions (13.5 percent) or were phrased in terms of "just" or "due" cause (54.7 percent).

TABLE 8.3

Distribution of Causes for Discharge Listed in
Hospital Contracts in the Tristate Area
and the United States, 1976
(in percentage of contracts)

Cause	Tristate Contracts (N = 126)	All U.S. Hospital Contracts (N = 817)
No provision	68.3	70.7
Unauthorized absence	20.6	18.7
Dishonesty or theft	7.9	5.8
Intoxication	6.3	4.9
Unauthorized work stoppage	6.3	4.8
Insubordination	5.6	4.3
Failure to obey safety rules	1.6	0.6
Incompetence	0.8	1.6
Misconduct	0.0	1.0
Other	9.5	7.6

Sources: Tristate contracts: Compiled by the authors. U.S. hospital contracts: Hervey A. Juris et al., "Employee Discipline No Longer Management Prerogative Only," Hospitals, JAHA 51 (May 1, 1977): 68.

As can be seen from the table, contract clauses specifying discharge for particular reasons do not differ greatly in frequency between the sample hospitals of the three states and the Juris sample of all hospitals. Second, in two-thirds of the contracts, any form of undesirable behavior may be grounds for involuntary termination; thus, hospital management generally has great leeway in the use of discharge. Third, a major surprise is that unauthorized absence would be the most frequently mentioned reason for discharge. Why so few contracts would specify dishonesty, intoxication, insubordination, or incompetence as reasons for discharge is unanswerable without additional data. One can only speculate that the parties to the labor agreements believed that a broad "due cause" clause would be understood to cover dishonesty and related transgressions. Unauthorized absence, however, may not customarily be considered as grounds for discharge and, therefore, must be specifically stated as such. Further, in an industry like the hospital, where turnover and absenteeism may be quite high and unauthorized absence a potential problem, a contract stipulation connecting absence and discharge may serve as a strong warning.

CONTRACTUAL RESTRAINTS ON LABOR UTILIZATION IN RETROSPECT

In reviewing the impact of collective bargaining on labor utilization in tristate area hospitals, it is clear that as of 1977 unions were placing very little restriction on the management of hospital manpower. Hospitals could subcontract, use supervisors for bargaining unit work, and assign individuals to tasks or machines without limitation. In addition, there were few contractual requirements to post jobs, provide training, or use seniority as the major or sole determinant in promotions, layoffs, or other personnel assignments. Although work rules initiated by the union may be a hindrance to productivity in such industries as construction, printing, or longshoring, that is not the case for the unionized hospitals of the three midwestern states investigated here. The impact of the labor agreement on hospital manpower administration is epitomized by the following contract clause taken from the labor agreement of a Wisconsin hospital:

The union further agrees that it will not directly or indirectly oppose or interfere with the legitimate and reasonable efforts of the hospital to maintain and improve the skill, efficiency, and ability of the employer or employee, and the union further agrees that

it will not in any manner oppose the installation of
new and improved methods of hospital administration. [20]

When union (or association) efforts to acquire, procedurally
and substantively, a voice in the management decisions of the area's
hospitals are considered, the evidence supports the conclusion of
both limited efforts and equally limited success. Few instances of
joint labor-management committees were uncovered outside the
public sector, since these would compel hospital administrators to
accept union control or codetermination of patient-care decisions.
The major exception was the continuing conflict arising among
nurses and housestaff over these concerns at Cook County hospitals
in Chicago.

The lack of labor-management controversy over work rules,
seniority, due process, staffing, or patient care in the hospitals of
Illinois, Minnesota, and Wisconsin can only be a matter of speculation. It may be a function of the health-care collective bargaining
climate prevailing in the three states. Other influences at work
may include such factors as the absence of militant leadership in
the various unions, both professional and nonprofessional, in the
region.

For groups such as registered nurses, licensure restricts
entrance to the occupations and sets rigid standards for professional
practice. [21] Restricted entry would enhance the economic position
of those who managed to get over the licensing hurdle as well as
reduce the need to protect one's "turf" through collective bargaining.

For all categories of hospital employees, the rapid expansion
of the industry after the end of World War II has, until recently,
enabled hospitals to avoid economic constraints. As large sums of
money were being pumped into the industry by public and private
health-care insurance programs, unions were able to escape the
dilemma faced by labor organizations in other sectors of the economy—that is, a choice between employment or wages. Both apparently were attainable in the hospital industry. As long as hospital
jobs were readily available and cost-pass-through mechanisms
operated, a confrontation between the needs of workers for job
security and of management for efficiency could be avoided.

Forces beyond the control of both employees and managers in
the hospitals of the region give indications of destabilizing the historical collective bargaining relationships. Labor law reforms,
cost containment programs, overbuilding of facilities, increasing
costs of technology, prospective surpluses of professionals, and
the drive for greater professional stature among RNs, housestaff,
and related employees together are approaching a critical con-
juncture. The likelihood of significant changes in the industrial

relations of hospitals will be examined in some detail in the conclud-
ing chapter of this report. First, however, there remains the
necessity of integrating the various dimensions of collective bargaining and hospital labor costs, which have been considered separately up to this point.

NOTES

1. Neil W. Chamberlain and Donald E. Cullen, The Labor
Sector, 2d ed. (New York: McGraw-Hill, 1971), p. 219.
2. Ibid. See also, Jack Barbash, "The Elements of Industrial Relations," British Journal of Industrial Relations 2 (March
1964): 66-78.
3. See Chapter 5.
4. Taft-Hartley Amendments: Implications for the Health
Care Field (Chicago: American Hospital Assocation, 1976), p. 11.
5. Health/Labor Management Report 3 (November 28,
1975): 1.
6. Health/Labor Management Report 5 (July 11, 1977): 4.
7. Health/Labor Management Report 3 (April 1, 1975): 1.
8. For illustrations, see the nursing strikes reported in
Health/Labor Relations Report 3 (November 28, 1975): 4; 4 (September 13, 1976): 3-4; and 5 (February 14, 1977): 3.
9. Howard L. Lewis, "Nurses: How Much Like Doctors?,"
Modern Health Care 3 (June 1975): 48-49.
10. Ibid., p. 49.
11. See Kathy Jianino, "Staffing, Patient Care, and Collective
Bargaining" (Paper presented at Federal Mediation and Conciliation
Service/Industrial Relations Research Association Meeting, Los
Angeles, November 1976), pp. 1-2.
12. Ibid.
13. Health/Labor Management Report 2 (July 1974): 3.
14. Ibid.
15. Hervey A. Juris, "Labor Agreements in the Hospital
Industry: A Study of Collective Bargaining Outputs," in Proceedings
of the 1977 Annual Spring Meeting of the Industrial Relations Research
Association, ed. Gerald G. Somers (Madison: Industrial Relations
Research Association, 1977), p. 511.
16. Taft-Hartley Amendments, p. 11.
17. Juris, "Labor Agreements," p. 507.
18. Ibid.
19. Hervey Juris et al., "Employee Discipline No Longer
Management Prerogative Only," Hospitals, JAHA 51 (May 1, 1977):
68.

20. Collective Bargaining Agreement between Local 150, Service Employees International Union, and LaCrosse (Wisconsin) Lutheran Hospital, 1975-1980.

21. Nathan Hershey, "Labor Relations in Hospitals in the Private Sector," in Proceedings of the Twenty-Second Annual Meeting of the Industrial Relations Research Association, ed. Gerald G. Somers (Madison: Industrial Relations Research Association, 1969), p. 217.

9

THE INFLUENCE OF COLLECTIVE BARGAINING ON HOSPITAL COSTS

Estimates of the collective bargaining effect on labor costs provided in Chapter 7 are an important first step in understanding its impact on the final cost of hospital services. It cannot necessarily be assumed, however, that a one-to-one ratio exists between changes in compensation and changes in the average cost per patient day. We should not even expect an effect equal to the ratio of labor costs to total costs, because labor costs are a product of price and quantity, and we have a measure only of the former. Moreover, it can be argued that collective bargaining influences the costs of operating an organization in many ways other than simply through employee compensation. Influences on a firm's internal labor market and employee turnover are other potential outcomes when a union is introduced into an organization.

A number of studies have considered the question of hospital cost functions in general, while others have dealt with the union effects on hospital wages in particular.[1] Among the former, work by Judith Lave and Lester Lave, Ralph Berry, and David Salkever, for example, is designed primarily to test hypotheses other than those relating to the impact of unions on costs. The latter studies, on the other hand, are limited to investigating only part of the potential effect of unions on costs and often draw upon data for years that do not adequately represent the situation in the mid-1970s, particularly in the wake of the recent amendments to the NLRA that have tended to strengthen unionism in the industry. (A discussion of these studies is contained in Chapter 7.)

Beyond the limited evidence on the union impact on wages, there are no empirical estimates of the likely union impact on non-wage costs or on hospital charges generally. In light of the many ways students of the labor movement suggest that collective bargaining influences the operation and rewards of an organization, the purpose of this chapter is to make an exploratory analysis of how several of these nonwage effects might supplement or offset the more commonly studied wage effect as a possible influence on hospital costs.

CONCEPTUAL FRAMEWORK

Hospital costs are essentially a function of the quantity and quality of services provided, the mix of services, factor costs, and efficiency. Although each of these dimensions is an important influence, this research is limited to the union effect on hospital costs; we will not attempt to fully specify a hospital cost function but will concentrate on providing sufficient specification to generate unbiased estimates of the union effects on these costs. Therefore, our discussion will focus on the limited area of the union impact on costs and will not include the more general analysis of hospital cost functions.[2]

When a hospital enters into a collective bargaining relationship, it faces two potential sources of union cost effects—changes in factor costs and efficiency. These influences stem from several sources. Beyond the likely impact of hospital wage rates noted previously, unions can also be expected to affect fringe benefits, perhaps to a greater extent than wages.[3] In light of the growing importance of fringe benefits in total compensation in all industries, these benefit effects could significantly influence total labor costs.

In addition to potentially higher compensation for labor, the hospital may also employ greater quantities of supervisory and administrative labor to carry out the terms of the contract. Particularly important might be the higher personnel department expenses associated with increased demands for record keeping and grievance and dispute settlement procedures. Similarly, hiring more sophisticated industrial relations staff may be required as well.[4]

Unionism can also affect efficiency, though these influences may be somewhat offsetting. For example, if work rules and job duties become more formalized under collective bargaining, existing staff may not be willing or able to perform as wide a range of tasks as they once did. As a result, the hospital may have to increase its personnel to maintain past levels of productivity. On the other hand, the introduction of a union and "industrial jurisprudence" to the organization is likely to improve efficiency by reducing employee turnover.[5] For example, in addition to improving wage and nonwage benefits, a strengthened seniority system, the hallmark of a unionized occupation, can reduce turnover in two ways. First, seniority makes organizational rewards contingent upon length of service and second, by providing an objective measure by which to allocate these rewards, introduces more equity into the workplace.[6]

In summary, the union represents potential costs (and savings) to the hospital, not only in terms of the financial gains that may accrue to its members but also as an institutional relationship that forces the hospital to reorganize its method of operation. While this latter influence can be translated into higher administrative costs, these may partially be offset by any savings derived from greater employee stability associated with unionism. The purpose of this chapter is to draw together evidence of the magnitude of these various union effects and provide an estimate of their net impact on hospital costs.

ESTIMATION MODEL

Labor Costs

Four variables are employed to determine the union influence on hospital costs. COMP is the average annual total compensation for an employee in the jth hospital. The variable is constructed by dividing total annual expenditures for wages and fringe benefits by the number of full-time-equivalent staff positions in the hospital (excluding interns, residents, and other trainees).[7] Clearly, the expected sign for COMP will be positive.

TO is the average annual rate of turnover in the jth hospital. The expectation is that while turnover may not be quite as costly for hospitals as for other organizations because of the general nature of many of the skills, the relationship between TO and hospital costs will still be positive. Including TO and COMP in the model will enable us to estimate the marginal cost of employee turnover and compensation.

The remaining effects of unionism are estimated in two ways. UH is a dummy variable representing the presence of a union in the hospital, while MU indicates the number of bargaining units in the jth hospital. MU represents multiple bargaining units within the hospitals, and the hypothesis tested is that fractional bargaining will lead to internal whipsawing and higher costs.

The estimation model and hypothesis will be as follows:

$$AC = c_0 + c_1 UH + c_2 MU + c_3 TO + c_4 COMP + c_5 Y$$
$$+ c_6 REL + c_7 GOVPER + c_8 SIZE + c_9 OCC + c_{10} TEACH$$
$$+ c_{11} POP + z_i. \tag{1}$$

$$c_1, c_2, c_3, c_4, c_5, c_7, c_{10}, c_{11} > 0; \quad c_6, c_9 < 0; \quad c_8 = ?$$

The coefficients on UH and MU will indicate the effects of unionism on hospital costs, independent of any union effect on compensation or turnover, and serve to represent the "institutional" costs of unionism. The figure below describes the relationship to be estimated.

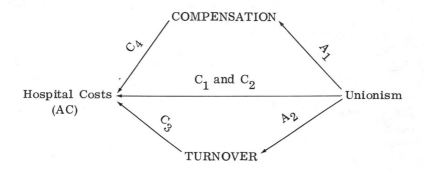

The effects identified by the c_i's correspond to the coefficients in Equation (1). In this framework unionism has a direct effect on hospital costs $(c_1 + c_2)$ that, it is argued, reflects the institutional impact of unionism. The indirect effects are represented as changes in COMP and TO that in turn affect AC. These indirect effects will be computed as

$$[(a_1 * \overline{COMP}) * c_4] \text{ and } [(a_2 * \overline{TO}) * c_3].^{\dagger}$$

The estimation of (a_1) and (a_2) are discussed below.

---

† To determine the unit change in TO or COMP that will be multiplied by (C_4), a_1 and a_2 must be converted from percentages to the appropriate units of measure. For convenience it was assumed that the most reasonable value would be the mean levels of the two variables defined as $\overline{COMP}$ and $\overline{TO}$. The estimation process is similar to a path model without resorting to standardized regression coefficients.

Control Variables

Several control variables in the model serve as proxies for variation in case mix. For example, hospital size (SIZE), measured by the number of beds, cribs, and pediatric bassinets regularly maintained by the hospital, is positively related to more expensive services, although economies of scale may offset this. By omitting an appropriate measure of case mix, the sign of SIZE will probably be positively biased. Therefore, although we will observe a biased effect for the size variable, the strong correlation between SIZE and case mix should prevent the union coefficients from being biased by this omission.[8]

For a similar reason, a dummy variable, TEACH, was included to denote whether the hospital was a member of the Council of Teaching Hospitals of the Association of American Medical Colleges. These hospitals typically offer the most sophisticated services requiring greater investments in technology and more highly skilled personnel; the result should be higher average costs, ceteris paribus. A measure of church operated hospitals (REL) is included as a dummy variable. Hospitals operated by religious orders tend to face more stringent budget constraints and as a result may attempt to reduce costs by seeking to lower factor prices. More importantly, because UH and REL are so highly correlated, c_1 could be biased if REL were omitted.[9] As a rough measure of hospital efficiency, we use average occupancy rate (OCC). OCC is defined as the ratio of the average daily census to the average number of beds maintained during the year. The expectation is that as occupancy rate expands (within a reasonable range) average costs will drop due to the relatively high ratio of fixed costs to total costs in the industry.

County population (POP) and median county income (Y) for 1970 will represent proxies for several variables. First, high income and urban areas should experience higher factor costs and thus pick up cost-of-living differences facing hospitals in different areas. Secondly, these variables are likely to represent areas of greater demand for hospital services and as a result higher costs. Because these are areas where unions are most organized, their omission would overstate the true union effects on hospital costs. While the levels of these variables have no doubt changed between 1970 and 1975, the assumption is that the distribution has been reasonably stable; that is, counties with relatively high incomes or population in 1970 also ranked among the top in 1975.

And finally, given the concern over the possible cost effects of a government administered health insurance system, the percent of third-party revenues derived from governmental sources (GOVPER) will be included as an independent variable. It is widely believed, for example, that hospitals are more easily able to pass on higher costs to government agencies than to private insurers.

DATA

The principal source of data for the analysis was the survey questionnaire discussed in Chapter 7. Short-term, general-care hospitals were selected as the unit of observation because they represent nearly 85 percent of all hospitals and have reasonably homogeneous organizational and service characteristics compared to long-term hospitals.

The data are characterized by the same response rate problems discussed in Chapter 7. As for the dependent variable, while the population and sample values were somewhat different, the margin was not dramatic.† Average cost per patient day was $133/day in the population compared to $127 in the sample. The most likely reason for the discrepancy was that Minnesota hospitals, which tend to be characterized by lower than average costs, were overrepresented in the sample.[10] Descriptive statistics and the data source for each variable in Equation 1 are reported in Table 9.1.

RESULTS

The dependent variable AC is the average cost per patient day in 1975. While log and semilog functions yielded similar effects, the arithmetic results will be presented because the estimates were more stable. (See Table 9.2.) With some interesting exceptions, the coefficients are reasonably stable and in the expected direction. Hospitals with one union have $6.42 higher average costs per patient day than nonunion hospitals, which is a difference of slightly more than 5 percent. The $6.42 figure is calculated by adding the coefficient of NU and UH together, when NU is evaluated at 1.00. This represents direct effect of unions on such hospital costs as grievance and dispute settlement procedures, changes in staffing patterns, and other institutional effects, and is above and beyond any impact on

---

†The final sample was 108 because missing observations had to be dropped. There was no significant difference, however, between this smaller group and the original 144 among the variables included in the regression model.

TABLE 9.1

Descriptive Statistics of Variables in Hospital Cost Functions

Variable	Mean	Standard Deviation
Average operating cost per patient day (AC)[a]	$126.72	33.63
Union hospital (UH)[a]	24.7	43.3
Number of bargaining units (MU)[a]	.619	1.358
Government reimbursement percent (GOVPER)[a]	47.2	14.2
Beds (SIZE)[b]	231.23	196.85
Occupancy rate (OCC)[b]	69.9	14.7
Teaching hospital (TEACH)[b]	7.1	25.7
Population (in thousands) (POP)[c]	1,238.8	2,135.9
Run by religious order (REL)[a]	23.9	42.8
Median county income (Y)[c]	$9,846.0	1,890.4
Average hospital turnover rate (TO)[a]	26.0	12.5
Average annual compensation per employee (COMP)[b]	$8,423.0	2,471.7

Note: Unless otherwise specified the figures are percentages.
Sources: a: Mailed questionnaire of hospitals, 1976.
b: Guide to the Health Care Field (Chicago: American Hospital Association, 1976).
c: U.S., Department of Health, Education, and Welfare, National Center for Health Statistics, Hospitals: A County and Metropolitan Area Data Book (Washington, D.C.: Government Printing Office, 1973).

TABLE 9.2

Regression Results of Hospital Cost Functions
(dependent variable: average cost per patient
day in the jth hospital [AC])

Independent Variables	
Constant	44.19
	(22.72)
Union hospital (UH)	9.772
	(8.91)
Number of bargaining units (NU)	-3.35
	(3.04)
Annual hospital turnover rate (TO)	54.93[a]
	(20.21)
Average compensation (COMP)	.0039[a]
	(.00116)
County income (Y)	.00485[a]
	(.00187)
Religious hospital (REL)	-4.48
	(5.79)
Government reimbursement (GOVPER)	-22.93
	(19.18)
Hospital size (SIZE)	-.0041
	(.0227)
Occupancy rate (OCC)	-6.457
	(19.395)
Teaching hospital (TEACH)	34.624[a]
	(13.559)
County population (POP)	.00195
	(.00127)
N	108
R^2	.5000
S.E.E.	$23.85

[a]Significant at .01 level.
[b]Significant at .05 level.
Note: The standard error of the regression coefficient is in parentheses.
Source: Compiled by the authors from mailed questionnaire.

compensation. While neither of the union coefficients is statistically significant at conventional levels and therefore should be interpreted with caution, they do represent practical significance and should not be disregarded out of hand.

The "one union" example is considered to be the most representative indication of the union presence in the hospital because the vast majority of multiunion hospitals are located in one area, Minneapolis. Moreover, the bargaining structure at the multi-employer level requires that each union bargain against a united management front of 20 to 30 hospitals; this, in turn, restricts internal whipsawing within the multiunion hospital. Thus, multiple bargaining units appear to lead to lower costs when in fact this may only be the case when a multiple employer bargaining structure can provide a countervailing power. Therefore, to focus on the more easily generalized results, the "union effect" is considered to be represented by the one-union hospital in this sample.

Turning to other variables in the model, the coefficient on COMP indicates that a $1,000 change in average annual compensation per hospital will result in a $4.00 change in average costs. Based on the respective means for AC and COMP, this yields an elasticity of .26.[11] In Chapter 7, it was estimated that unions affect average hourly compensation (wages and fringe benefits) in the neighborhood of 5 percent among the hospitals in this sample. Given the compensation elasticity of .26, we can conclude that this increase in the level of compensation will have a small upward influence on average costs—on the order of 1.3 percent. By combining the two union effects, it seems that unions apparently increase average costs by a little more than 6 percent.

However, we must also examine how unions affect turnover and thereby offer potential savings to hospitals. The results in Table 9.2 indicate that, in fact, turnover is very expensive for hospitals. A one-standard deviation (.125) in the average annual turnover rate of hospitals would decrease average costs per patient day by nearly $7.00, or 5.4 percent. The importance of this relationship is underscored by the results of other analysis on these data, which suggest that for a sample of service workers, unionized occupations experience a 50 percent lower turnover than nonunionized groups.[12] Because unions may not necessarily influence the employment stability of all occupational groups to the same extent, a conservative assumption would be that an average effect (across all occupations) might be in the range of 20 to 30 percent. This would translate into a 2.2 to 3.5 percent decrease in AC.

Taken together, the three union effects suggest that, overall, union hospitals in the three states studied have experienced 2 to 4 percent higher average costs than nonunion hospitals. While these

magnitudes are not trivial, they do not support the argument that
labor unions have played a major role in the recent spiral of hospital
prices.

The results of the remaining variables were generally in the
expected direction and will be noted briefly. The sign of GOVPER
indicates that hospitals receiving greater percentages of their third-
party payments from governmental sources experience lower costs.
This result has been observed in other studies[13] and may be attrib-
utable to the fact that governmental reimbursements generally go to
hospitals in poorer areas. Clients there may be using the hospital
for basic medical care in lieu of a private physician, and, in all
likelihood, a higher portion of the clients may be elderly, requiring
longer average stays. In the first case, the product is relatively
inexpensive, and in the second, average costs are reduced by the
increased quantity of the service being utilized. The effect is that
we observe higher third-party payments by government insurers
(GOVPER) in lower cost hospitals. As a result, the actual effect
of larger percentages of government revenue is not really clear
from these data.

The insignificant negative sign on SIZE supports our earlier
hypothesis that this variable will pick up conflicting effects of case
mix and economies of scale. The remaining variables are in the
expected direction, though not always significant at conventional
levels.

SUMMARY AND CONCLUSION

Given the level of detail available from the survey data, this
analysis has provided a unique opportunity to measure the totality
of union effects on product costs, an issue that has not been well
studied in any industry. Unfortunately, to obtain these estimates
we have had to accept the qualitative limitations of the data in terms
of measurement error and potential nonresponse bias; therefore,
the study should be considered a first step.

These results provide support for the notion that unions can
have a variety of effects on organizational efficiency, some of
which may partially offset each other. Unions apparently have both
a positive and negative effect on hospitals' costs, the least significant of which is their influence on compensation. Though the estimates of the institutional effects must be viewed with caution, it
seems that unions impose certain fixed costs on hospitals by way of
organizational changes and added personnel expenses that tend to
exceed the direct costs of union compensation. However, as part
of this institutional change, labor unions also introduce "industrial

jurisprudence," which, along with other benefits, reduces employee turnover and, in turn, offers important savings to the organization. The net result of the competing influeu_es is slightly higher (2 to 4 percent) average costs in unionized hospitals.

Despite these caveats and the data limitations already discussed, this analysis provides little support for the argument that unions are a major source of the recent rise in hospital costs. Had the effects been even twice as large, the contribution of collective bargaining to past changes in the cost of hospital care would have been quite small simply because of the modest growth of unionism in the industry. The estimates reported here are roughly equivalent to comparing differences in hospital costs where the industry is 100 percent organized as opposed to it having no organization. Since the percentage of hospitals with collective bargaining contracts has increased from approximately 10 percent to 25 percent in recent years, the change in the industrywide average cost per patient day that can be attributed to the union sector remains quite small. Moreover, given our analysis of the hospital labor movement in the Midwest and other areas, there seems to be little reason to expect this pattern to change in the near future.

NOTES

1. See, for example, Judith R. Lave and Lester B. Lave, "Estimated Cost Functions for Pennsylvania Hospitals," Inquiry 8 (June 1970); 3-14; Ralph Berry, Jr., "Product Heterogeneity and Hospital Cost Analysis," Inquiry 8 (March 1970): 67-75; David S. Salkever, "A Micro-Economic Study of Hospital Cost Inflation," Journal of Political Economy 80 (November/December 1972): 1144-66; Martin Feldstein, Rising Cost of Hospital Care (Washington, D.C.: Information Resources Press, 1971); and Amy Kriger Taylor, "The Demand for Labor in Nonprofit Institutions: Studies of the Hospital Industry" (Ph.D. diss., Harvard University, 1974).

2. For a more thorough presentation on the general question of estimating hospital cost functions, see Martin Feldstein, "Hospital Cost Inflation," American Economic Review 61 (December 1971): 853-73.

3. Several reasons why the union effect on fringe benefits may be expected to exceed the union wage effect are provided in Bevars Mabry, "The Economics of Fringe Benefits," Industrial Relations 12 (February 1973): 95-106; and Albert Rees, "Some Non-Wage Aspects of Collective Bargaining," in The Public Stake in Union Power, ed. Phillip Bradley (Charlottesville: University of Virginia Press, 1959), pp. 124-43.

4. The classic reference to these and other institutional effects by unions is Sumner H. Slichter, James J. Healey, and Robert E. Livernash, The Impact of Collective Bargaining on Management (Washington, D. C.: Brookings Institution, 1960).

5. It has long been argued that the costs of unionization are overstated if, in fact, unions provide a stabilizing influence on the work force that in turn reduces turnover costs. These union influences on employee stability are discussed in Joseph Shister, "The Institutional Aspects of Mobility," in Proceedings of the Third Annual Winter Meeting of the Industrial Relations Research Association, ed. Milton Derber (Madison: Industrial Relations Research Association, 1950), pp. 42-59; while empirical support for these effects is provided in John H. Pencavel, An Analysis of the Quit Rate in American Manufacturing Industry (Princeton University, 1970).

6. Charles S. Telly, Wendell L. French, and William G. Scott, "The Relationship of Inequality to Turnover Among Hourly Workers," Administrative Science Quarterly 16 (June 1971): 164-72, offers some empirical support for the notion that equity considerations influence employee stability.

7. The total expenditures on wages and fringe benefits were computed from the mailed survey. Data on full-time-equivalent staff were obtained from Guide to the Health Care Field (Chicago: American Hospital Association, 1976).

8. While the measurement of case mix differences across hospitals has typically been a problem in the accurate specification of hospital cost functions, Lave and Lave, "Cost Functions," p. 14, found that the simple correlation between hospital size and their measure of case mix to be .76. Moreover, there is probably little reason to believe that unionism and case mix are correlated to any great extent, other than through the influence of hospital size on both variables.

9. It was felt that because unionism is so negatively correlated with REL, if AC were also correlated with REL c_1 would be biased. Hervey Juris et al., "Nationwide Survey Shows Growth in Union Contracts," Hospitals, JAHA 51 (March 16, 1977): 125, table 1 suggests that nationally less than 1 percent of church-affiliated hospitals are organized.

10. The population values were calculated from Hospital Statistics (Chicago: American Hospital Association, 1976), table 5C. The concern with the dependent variable is really that the conditional distribution of AC be representative. That is, if hospitals of equal size, case mix, and so forth, systematically responded differently so that only low or high cost hospitals were included in the sample, then the regression coefficients would be biased. However,

there is no reason to believe that this might occur a priori and given the variance in AC this does not appear to be a problem.

11. While labor costs make up between 50 and 60 percent of total costs, these figures include both the price of labor and the quantity employed. The .26 estimate reflects the impact of changes in only the price of labor and is consistent with recent results reported in Martin Feldstein and Amy Kriger Taylor, The Rapid Rise of Hospital Costs (Washington, D.C.: Council on Wage and Price Stability, 1977), pp. 13-19.

12. See Brian Becker, "Hospital Unionism and Employment Stability," Industrial Relations 17 (February 1978): 96-101, for a discussion of this analysis. Union effects of a similar magnitude are reported for manufacturing industries in Pencavel, Quit Rate.

13. Salkever, "Hospital Cost Inflation," pp. 1157-58.

10

CONCLUSIONS

The preceding chapters have presented a picture of an industry undergoing rapid and far-reaching changes in both structure and operation. The continuing advances of medical science have made obsolete the long-term care hospital and are radically modifying the form of the short-term. The number of outpatient visits is increasing rapidly, as is the number of empty hospital beds. New technology is revolutionizing diagnosis and treatment, but necessitates vast and burdensome capital expenditures.

Not the least of the recent developments for hospitals has been the advent of private and public insurance programs that have effectively removed the patient as the direct source of a health-care institution's revenue. Medicare, Medicaid, Blue Cross-Blue Shield, and related programs have injected billions of dollars into the industry, much of it within the past ten years. While the funds have provided the means by which the delivery of medical services could be greatly expanded and improved, they have also been a mechanism for outside control of all phases of the hospital industry from construction to operation. Moreover, the growing influence of third parties not affiliated with health care has been reinforced by widespread concern over the current and especially the future expense of health-care programs. The automatic pass-through of costs is being replaced by systems of prospective reimbursement. A threat also exists in the imposition by the federal government of an absolute upper limit on the increase in hospital costs; however they are yet to be determined.

As a consequence of all of these changes, a number of trends in the industry are already discernible. First, hospitals are becoming larger and more bureaucratically structured. Second, a shift in services provided is occurring as long-term care declines

141

and short-visit, outpatient treatment becomes important. Third, in the face of debt burdens and cost constraints, hospitals are closing, merging, or sharing technology, departments, and services.

These trends have had direct repercussions on the labor market of the industry as well as on the work forces of individual hospitals. Total employment has grown rapidly, as has the average number of employees per hospital and per bed. With the new technology and treatment, specialized employees, particularly at the professional level, have become characteristic of the modern urban hospital. In addition, the proportion of part-time and voluntary workers has diminished. Finally, the compensation of hospital employees has climbed markedly.

Like many service industries, health care generally and hospitals in particular have historically experienced a low incidence of unionization among their employees. Collective bargaining has been concentrated in certain geographical areas of the United States and has been primarily confined to the large, urban, nonreligious hospital. The limited extent of hospital unions is a consequence of many factors, but a key has been the exclusion of private, nonprofit hospitals from the coverage of the federal labor relations law. With the removal of that exclusion in 1974, in theory at least, a spur to the growth of collective bargaining in hospitals has been provided.

HOSPITAL LABOR RELATIONS IN ILLINOIS, MINNESOTA, AND WISCONSIN

The hospitals in the tristate area have not been insulated from either the general trends in the industry or from those that concern labor relations directly. The impact, however, was different in each state. Minnesota already possessed an extensive framework for hospital collective bargaining that, while protecting union organizing, substituted compulsory arbitration for the right to strike. Its health-care labor force, both professional and nonprofessional, was well-organized before the decade of the 1950s ended, and thus, by 1974, hospital collective bargaining was quite stable and free of conflict.

Illinois, on the other hand, had no legal framework for hospital labor relations, and the result was a system in which force at times was the primary arbiter of disagreement between labor and management. The potential for calamitous consequences in both recognition and negotiation disputes persuaded the parties to establish a series of preelection agreements to fill the void created by the lack of a formal legal structure. Under the circumstances, conflict often was intense, higher than in either of the other two states, and collective bargaining remained largely a phenomenon localized in Chicago.

Wisconsin, for its part, exhibited characteristics of both Illinois and Minnesota. Although it possessed a statutory system providing for recognition, bargaining, and the right to strike, its level of unionization in hospitals did not reach that of Minnesota. Moreover, the conflict level in Wisconsin, while not as high as that of Illinois, nevertheless significantly exceeded that of Minnesota.

Another important difference between the three states is in the structure of bargaining. In Illinois and Wisconsin, hospitals bargain separately, although they do so at times with the assistance of local hospital councils. Minnesota's structure, on the other hand, is centered in multihospital negotiating units, sometimes covering as many as 20 or more organizations. In addition, Minnesota hospitals are likely to be faced with fragmented multiple bargaining units among their employees. Separate contracts occur frequently for such groups as RNs, LPNs, pharmacists, radiologic technologists, and power plant personnel, among others. These occupations tend not to be represented for collective bargaining outside of Minnesota; hence, hospitals in the three states usually bargain with only a nonprofessional union representing a service employees unit. If additional unions are present in any one hospital, it is most frequently a local of the Operating Engineers acting on behalf of power plant workers.

The third-party payer, a major element in the hospital bargaining structure in such areas as the northeastern United States, is missing from the tristate area. Although rate review commissions and other forms of fiscal control exist, they have not yet become a factor in bargaining outcomes. As will be discussed below, this situation is one of several aspects of hospital labor relations in the Midwest that will very likely change.

Finally, it should be noted that the impact of collective bargaining goes significantly beyond the immediate parties involved. In the first place, pattern bargaining is characteristic of Illinois, Wisconsin, and Minnesota hospitals, with the result that key settlements become the reference points for many other negotiations. Second, there is evidence that spillover, threat, or ripple effects extend terms to the nonunionized employees and hospitals in the three states. Thus, "orbits of coercive comparison" were found to encompass union and nonunion hospitals alike.

IMPACT OF THE 1974 AMENDMENTS

Unlike those in many other parts of the United States, labor organizations in the tristate area were a going concern when private, nonprofit hospitals came under the jurisdiction of federal labor law. The relative absence of conflict over recognition, rights, or interests is an indication that collective bargaining relations were mature and peaceful, as, in fact, they had been before the end of the 1960s. Thus, it is not surprising that, for the most part, the 1974 amendments did not provide a stimulus to unionization of the industry. Further, to the degree that the amendments removed the possibility of using strikes to achieve recognition, they may have introduced handicaps.

In addition, the board of inquiry scheme that Congress devised for resolving impasses has not been a factor in hospital bargaining in the three states. There already was little inclination to use strikes or job actions, and, in significant instances in Minnesota and Illinois, the parties had committed themselves to arbitration should negotiations break down.

IMPACT OF COLLECTIVE BARGAINING ON
HEALTH-CARE ADMINISTRATION

A major objective of our study was to assess the extent to which collective bargaining has positive or negative consequences for the cost and efficiency of the delivery of health care. Among the questions addressed were: (1) Does collective bargaining raise the compensation of hospital employees and, if so, by how much? (2) Does collective bargaining place constraints on hospital management's use of its labor force? (3) Does collective bargaining raise hospital costs and, if so, by how much? (4) Is the delivery of health care subject to interruptions and, if so, what kind and of what duration?

Answers to these questions were sought through data collected on short-term community hospitals of Illinois, Minnesota, and Wisconsin. Field interviews were employed, a questionnaire was mailed to each of the 563 community hospitals in the three states, and secondary sources were searched for relevant information. In addition, an analysis of 126 hospital labor contracts from the area was undertaken with the assistance of the American Hospital Association.

COLLECTIVE BARGAINING AND
HOSPITAL COMPENSATION

Our analysis of changes in both wages and fringe benefits under unionization provides evidence that, on the average, unions did in

fact tend to raise occupational wages on the order of 5 percent.
This estimate stems from the direct effect on unionized occupations
as well as the spillover effect on nonunion occupations in unionized
hospitals.

There are several reasons why it is not surprising that these
effects are below those reported for other unionized industries,
especially manufacturing. First, given the labor intensity of the
industry, we would expect greater management resistance to union
wage demands. Second, the institutional analysis suggests that
hospital unions in the three states have not been particularly militant in bargaining.

The union effect on fringe benefits averaged nearly 11 percent.
Because few other studies have addressed the union effect on benefits, we have little evidence with which to compare these results.
Here, too, there are several reasons why the union impact on
fringe benefits would exceed that on wages. First, in the face of
strong management opposition to direct wage increases, leaders of
relatively weak unions may have to settle for benefits as the major
ingredient of the economic part of a settlement package. Second,
benefits may be appealing to management in a high turnover industry
such as the hospital, since many employees may leave before col-
lecting benefits. Finally, if payment is made, it is often delayed,
and thus the real cost to management may be much lower than direct
wage or salary costs.

COLLECTIVE BARGAINING AND
LABOR UTILIZATION

Our analysis of hospital labor agreements collected in the
three states, supplemented by field interviews and the questionnaire
survey, revealed that traditional controls over work rules and job
security often present in industrial labor-management agreements
are absent from health-care contracts. Very little restriction, if
any, is placed on management in the way it uses hospital manpower.
Hospitals can subcontract, unilaterally determine job content, use
supervisors for bargaining unit work, and assign whatever number
of individuals they deem appropriate to a task or machine.

More than half of the contracts analyzed had long probationary
periods (three months or more), 77 percent provided for no formal
training for promotion, and the use of length of service for upgrading or lateral movements was often a secondary consideration.

While the above generalizations hold for both professional and
nonprofessional labor agreements, there was an additional consideration for the former. Professionals in hospital work have often

pursued objectives related to participation in and/or control of patient-care decisions. Contracts examined and disputes investigated indicate that, for the most part, professionals employed in the private hospitals of Wisconsin, Illinois, and Minnesota have neither sought nor achieved a direct voice in patient-care issues.

In summary the impact of collective bargaining on manpower utilization in hospitals of the tristate area is minimal, and hospital administrators' fear that unionization would substantially reduce their discretion has not been realized.

COLLECTIVE BARGAINING AND HOSPITAL COSTS

Health care is an industry in which labor costs constitute 50 to 60 percent of total costs. It is also an industry in which the cost of health care to the consumer is rising at a much faster rate than prices in other sectors of the economy. Therefore, we believed that it was important to determine if union effects on compensation are influencing the cost of hospital care, and if so, to what extent. We also wanted to find out if there were any indirect union influences on costs. For example, did the presence of unions in a hospital reduce employee turnover, thus creating savings for the hospital? Or, what additional costs, if any, might be incurred through the establishment of grievance and dispute settlement procedures, increased supervision, changes in staffing patterns, added demands on the personnel department, and the institutionalizing of the collective bargaining relationship?

To arrive at these estimates, we calculated the marginal effects of unionism, turnover, and compensation on average cost per patient day for the hospitals in our sample. First, unionized hospitals apparently experience approximately 5 percent higher costs from the union effect on grievance procedures, personnel practices, and so forth. Second, the effect on compensation (wages and fringe benefits) in turn led to 1.3 percent higher average costs in unionized hospitals.

Although these two influences tend to increase costs, unionized hospital occupations tend to experience up to 50 percent lower turnover than their nonunion counterparts. In light of the marginal cost of turnover, estimated from the hospital cost model, we calculated that unionized hospitals will have 2 to 4 percent lower average costs due to savings from lower turnover.

The net result of these three effects is an increase in average costs on the order of 2 to 4 percent. While these results do not represent a national sample, they do indicate that unions are probably not going to be a major source of hospital inflation in the near future.

COLLECTIVE BARGAINING AND THE
DELIVERY OF HEALTH CARE

The disruption of health-care services is, perhaps, the most feared outcome of collective bargaining by all concerned: union leaders, hospital administrators, government officials, and the general public. Opposition to unionization has, in fact, been rationalized through the argument that recognition of a union was an invitation to strike. Job actions, picket lines, and work stoppages would not only cause great inconvenience but also endanger the health and safety of patients.

The desire of hospital labor and management to ensure that health services continue in the event of disputes is reflected in many ways in the three states in our sample. First, the level of conflict is generally lower for the hospital industry than for other types of service or manufacturing activities. Second, the parties have willingly accepted the use of arbitration for impasse resolution and, at times, voluntarily given up the right to strike. Third, when strikes have occurred, there is no evidence that hospitals have been completely shut down. Patients are transferred; supervisors and volunteers continue working; and other employees, including members of other unions in the hospital, cross picket lines.

The absence of conflict in hospital labor relations is a consequence of many factors, not all of which exist in each state to the same degree. Such factors as social climate are important in Minnesota generally and in the smaller cities and rural areas of Wisconsin and Illinois. Across the three states, the major unions or associations have faced little competition from rival unions, and officers have had few challenges to their leadership. The long period of compulsory arbitration under the Charitable Hospitals Act seems to have conditioned the parties in Minnesota to look beyond the strike to more amicable systems of dispute settlement. Whatever the reasons, up to 1977 union recognition has not been an invitation to the disruption of medical services.

In summing up the impact of collective bargaining, one is at first tempted to conclude that the effects have been negligible. But this would not be an accurate accounting of the changes that have come in the wake of the first stages of unionization of the hospital industry. Part of the problem of measuring the extent to which wages and costs are higher in unionized hospitals is that nonunion employees in hospitals with or without union contracts almost immediately are granted the benefits accepted in contract settlements. Whether because of spillover or threat, wages in nonunion situations may equal or exceed those of workers under labor agreements, grievance systems come into existence, and supervisors receive training in human relations and related subjects. Moreover, the general personnel management function may be significantly upgraded in both budget and status.[1]

When labor disputes have occurred in the hospitals of the tristate area, they historically have arisen in conjunction with union-organizing drives. Once the employees' organization was recognized, conflict usually diminished, and, with the "threat" removed, the pressures to keep compensation and job conditions in advance of the unionized health-care sector were no longer compelling. Thus, it is ironic that the impact of collective bargaining, at least in the short run, may have been greatest on nonunion hospitals.

THE FUTURE OF HOSPITAL LABOR RELATIONS
IN ILLINOIS, WISCONSIN, AND MINNESOTA

In the immediate future, the basic structure and climate for health-care collective bargaining in the three states will not change radically. The number of new bargaining units being organized is small, the existing labor organizations are well entrenched, and the relations between the parties have been positive. Left to their own devices, labor and management would expand collective bargaining in a very gradual fashion and, likely, without a great deal of conflict.

Unfortunately for the long-term stability of hospital labor relations, external pressures that will force major changes in collective bargaining are rapidly gathering momentum. Those most identifiable at the moment seem to be the following: First, outside fiscal and capital control has been only of marginal concern to the negotiators in hospitals. Unlike those in the northeastern United States, third-party payers in the tristate area have not intruded on the bargaining process. It is clear, however, that this situation is nearly at an end. Each of the three states is moving toward mandatory review and control of nearly all phases of hospital administration. The replacement of cost-pass-through reimbursement with prospective reimbursement alters the nature of the settlement process. Finally, the overriding concern with the cost of publicly financed health-care programs makes legislated cost ceilings a strong probability.

The onus, thus, is on hospital management to cut costs, generate savings, and improve its efficiency in any way possible. For labor, the consequences are obvious. Workers will be laid off or terminated permanently as hospitals close, departments merge, and services are shared or subcontracted. In the face of a probable surplus of professionals and continuing high levels of urban minority unemployment, the clash between job security and management efficiency, which has been muted until now, will emerge as a major factor separating the parties. With compensation already relatively low in the industry, the likelihood is that efforts to reduce the wage differentials that exist between health-care and other industries will face further barriers. This fact, too, will exacerbate the fiscal problems that will be associated with demands for job security.

A second factor that has implications for the current configuration of hospital collective bargaining involves the social values most closely associated with female work roles. Given the high proportion of women in the health-care labor market, changes in their attitudes and perceptions toward labor force participation, joining unions, activism, or conflict in confrontation with male hospital authority figures all can have important consequences for labor relations in hospitals. When it is no longer considered unprofessional, undignified, or unladylike to contest grievances, march on picket lines, or engage in job actions, the militance of the industry's labor organizations will rise accordingly. Moreover, the demonstration effect produced by the collective action of other professionals such as teachers, a high proportion of whom are women, will reinforce these tendencies.

A final factor, also associated with the change of social values, is the likelihood that pressures will mount among hospital professionals in the tristate area to obtain a greater voice in patient care decisions. The die has already been cast at the national level by such groups as the American Nurses Association and at the local level by the action of state associations in Ohio, Connecticut, California, and Illinois.

In the first place, the long-held belief that a contradiction exists between professionalism and collective bargaining is being discarded. Health-care professionals have begun to accept the conclusion that "collective bargaining can be an effective process for bringing about a redistribution of the base of power within the health service organization."[2]

The attainment of control of practice is viewed positively by professionals for various reasons. On the one hand, they feel it will give them an opportunity to make significant gains for patient welfare.[3] On the other hand, the attainment of professional control is seen as a means by which the status of the profession can be raised.[4] "Only by working collectively to define and enforce standards of care will nursing be able to gain the public's recognition of the value of its services and its entitlement to greater personal reward. The negotiated contract can become a legal means to hold nursing and hospital administration accountable."[5]

Although professional control issues have not had high salience in the private hospitals in our study, the external forces at work on health care may very well bring it to the front as a collective bargaining issue. As pointed out, patient-care considerations may become a direct challenge to management as well as have implications for staffing, job assignments, and other cost-related decisions. Forces beyond the control of both the hospital manager and the professional employee are pulling the parties onto a collision course.

Labor relations in the hospital industry of Illinois, Wisconsin, and Minnesota seem to be entering a transitional phase. The next phase will likely be marked by higher levels of conflict than witnessed previously and a general uncertainty as new relationships and structures are created. In the long run, hospital collective bargaining in the tristate area may again function in a peaceful and efficient manner. This, too, appears to be an outcome largely beyond the control of the parties.

NOTES

1. See Phyllis Greenberg, "Influence of the Taft-Hartley Amendment on Health Care Facilities," (Unpublished paper, University of Wisconsin—Madison, December 1975), p. 13; and Anthony Robbins, "Professionalism and the Power of Management in Health Services," in Proceedings of the Twenty-Third Annual Winter Meeting of the Industrial Relations Research Association, ed. Gerald G. Somers (Madison: Industrial Relations Research Association, 1971), pp. 146-52.

2. Virginia Cleland, "Taft-Hartley Amended: Implications for Nursing—The Professional Model," American Journal of Nursing (February 1975): 288.

3. Ibid. Also, Ingeborg G. Mauksch, "Attainment of Control Over Professional Practice," Nursing Forum 10 (1971): 233-38.

4. Ada Jacox, "Collective Action and Control of Practice by Professionals," Nursing Forum 10 (1971): 239-57.

5. Cleland, "Taft-Hartley Amended," p. 289.

APPENDIX:

THE ENDOGENEITY OF WAGES, UNIONISM, AND TURNOVER

As we suggested in Chapter 7, it may be that unionism, wages, and turnover are best described by a model in which all three variables are considered endogenous.[1] If, in fact, they are endogenous and the union effect is estimated in a single equation model, it will be positively biased and overstate the union impact on relative wages. To resolve this problem, these relationships will be estimated using two-stage least squares (2SLS), which provide consistent estimates for overidentified systems as well as a degree of convenience.

The service workers will be used as the only sample group for several reasons. First, this group provides the most consistent and stable estimates of a positive union effect on wages. Therefore, we will not be faced with the potential interpretative problems of comparing two "insignificant" coefficients. Second, this group offers the largest sample size; this is important because we must drop missing values for most variables in all three equations in order to estimate the wage equation. And, finally, because of the relatively large union effect (compared to other groups), it is of some policy interest to know if, in fact, this is a "true" estimate and not a potentially biased one.

Table A.1 presents the comparable results for ordinary least squares (OLS) and 2SLS when a wage model is employed that can be more easily compared to those of other studies (that is, no NU * UH variable is present). As is consistent with the hypothesis in Chapter 7, the 2SLS estimate does show a much smaller union effect on wages. The 2SLS coefficient indicates that a union member will only receive a .6 percent relative wage differential compared to a 5 percent effect in a comparably specified OLS model. It should also be noted that the estimate is very unstable and could not be accepted as different from zero within conventional confidence limits.

TABLE A.1

Comparison of OLS and 2SLS Wage Regressions
for Service Workers
(dependent variable: natural logarithm of
average hourly money wage rate)

Independent Variables	OLS	2SLS
Constant	.6056[a]	.6789[a]
	(.0519)	(.1174)
Union member U	.0481[a]	.00646
	(.0141)	(.08901)
Percent turnover	-.0078	-.7924
	(.0286)	(.5942)
Percent female	.0552[b]	-.06947
	(.02645)	(.1123)
Percent minority	.0126	.003243
	(.0254)	(.04154)
Government reimbursements	-.0747[c]	-.03733
	(.0402)	(.0790)
Median county income	.000036[a]	.000054[a]
	(.0000037)	(.0000126)
Beds	.00027[a]	.000408[a]
	(.000044)	(.000148)
Teaching hospital	-.0609[b]	-.1236[b]
	(.0293)	(.0585)
Population in country	.000029[a]	.000029[a]
	(.0000029)	(.00000469)
Beds/total beds in country	.00253	.01107
	(.00695)	(.01468)
N	506	495
$\overline{R}^2$	.6045	—d

[a]Significant at .01 level.
[b]Significant at .05 level.
[c]Significant at .10 level.
d$\overline{R}^2$ not available for 2SLS.

Note: The standard error of the regression coefficient is in parentheses.

Source: Compiled by the authors from mailed questionnaire.

While the conclusion with respect to the bias of the single equation model will not be affected, we should point out that the 2SLS is to some extent biased toward zero as a result of the estimation procedure employed. Specifically, since 2SLS uses predicted values of the endogenous variables (unionism and turnover), the union variable represents a dichotomous variable being predicted by a least squares technique. Among other problems, some of the predicted values tend to fall outside the zero-to-one bound and, in general, are biased estimates as these bounds are approached.† Therefore, for high and low values of U, the measurement error is increased. However, since the total bias in B depends on the ratio of the variance of the error to the variance of the true value, the total effect of the bias is reasonably small because the error variance probably represents no more than 10 to 15 percent of the total variance in the union variable. Again, the magnitude of this bias is not enough to change our original conclusion.

As for the effect of turnover on the wages of service workers, the results in the 2SLS lend a little more support to the originally hypothesized negative relationship, although the estimate is only marginally significant at the .18 level. However, the direction of the change in the coefficient is unexpected. It suggests (and is supported by the 2SLS results of the turnover model) that the high wage workers have a higher turnover rate than low wage workers, ceteris paribus.†† While this is an apparent contradiction of the expected relationship, the a priori hypothesis is based on the assumption that higher wages mean "higher" compared to other opportunities in the labor market. Unfortunately, we have no information about the alternate wages available to the workers in the five occupations that compose the service worker sample. It is certainly conceivable that the ward clerks and switchboard operators who average $3.23 per hour would have better nonhospital alternatives than nurse's aides, kitchen helpers, and maids who average between $2.95 and $3.00 per hour. It is not unlikely that the

---

†U is now a continuous variable and not a zero-to-one dichotomous variable, because it is the predicted value of the original union member variable. However, if the U is evaluated at 1.00 and 0.0, the results can be interpreted as they are in the OLS model. We should also point out that no $\overline{R}^2$ is available from the 2SLS program, but given the significant levels of many of the coefficients, we might assume the entire equation to be significant at more than a .01 level.

††We draw this conclusion from the direction of the bias suggested by the change in the magnitude of the coefficient.

clerical and office skills possessed by the high wage group would be of use to a larger number of potential employers than the skills of a nurse's aide or maid.

Because the focus of this discussion is to note any change in the union coefficient in the wage model, it is not necessary to dwell on the various other coefficients and how they may or may not have been affected. However, we will briefly review the results of the other two equations in the system concerning the endogenous variables under investigation (unionism and turnover). Tables A.2 and A.3 include the results for the endogenous variables of interest.†

First, consider the impact of wages on the likelihood of being a union member. The prevailing opinion is that high wage workers are probably more likely to join a union because they are more interested in the conditions of work, and so forth, and probably demand more in services. Similarly, unions supply more services to high wage workers because of the greater financial returns. The OLS model appears to support this analysis. However, it may also be that low wage workers feel a greater need for union services and, with this greater demand, are able to more than overcome any union unwillingness to organize them. The results of the 2SLS equation indicate that this apparently may be the more accurate analysis.

The OLS model indicates that a \$1.00 increase in wages would be reflected in a 10 percent increase in the likelihood of union coverage, while the 2SLS results suggest that a \$1.00 increase in wages (approximately 32 percent of the \$3.09 mean) would <u>decrease</u> this same likelihood by a little more than 14 percent. While the 2SLS estimate is apparently so unreliable that we cannot reject the hypothesis that it is really equal to zero in the population, there is some uncertainty attached to this "insignificance" since we are using a dichotomous dependent variable and potentially biased standard errors.

---

†The exogenous variables in the unionism model were percent female in occupation, percent minority in occupation, hospital size, the existence of state labor legislation covering hospital workers, religious affiliation of hospital, and county population.

The exogenous variables in the turnover model included fringe benefit level, hospital size, percent female in occupation, percent minority in occupation, estimate of whether a labor shortage exists in occupation, upgrading available in occupation, number of other hospitals in county, and hospital size/total beds in county.

TABLE A.2

Partial Results of Unionism Model
(dependent variable: if the ith occupation is covered
by a collective bargaining agreement)

Independent Variables	OLS	2SLS
Constant	.0242	.2574
	(.1127)	(.2514)
Average wage	.1057[a]	-.4533
	(.0339)	(.4341)
Percent turnover	.1123	1.227
	(.0837)	(1.111)
N	639	495
$\overline{R}^2$	.1964	—[b]

[a]Significant at .01 level.

[b]$\overline{R}^2$ not available for 2SLS.

Notes: In the 2SLS models, wage is measured as lnW rather than W as in the OLS model. As a result, the interpretation of the coefficient will depend on the point from which the unit change in W occurs (that is, $\frac{\partial u}{\partial x} = \frac{B}{W}$). If the change in $1.00 is evaluated from

the mean of W—$3.00—then the change in u would be $\frac{(-.4533)}{3.60} = .14$.

The standard error of the regression coefficient is in parentheses.

Source: Compiled by the authors from mailed questionnaire.

Similarly, the effect of turnover on likelihood of unionism is contrary to our expected results. Both the OLS and 2SLS results suggest a positive relationship between turnover and unionism, although neither is significant by conventional standards. Once again, this result is certainly not implausible. It is generally argued that turnover primarily affects the supply of union services and that unions do not want to absorb the "costs" of high turnover workers. However, it should also be pointed out that certain unions may be willing to organize service workers regardless of these added costs because of concerns other than those simply financial in nature. In addition, as in the case of low wage workers, the higher turnover rates may reflect such unfavorable working conditions that the demand for union services is significantly increased, with the net effect being more union membership. This process would be further reinforced if unions were able to reduce turnover after organization and, therefore, capture the advantages of worker stability anyway. As we will see, this, in fact, has been the case. The tenfold increase in the magnitude of the turnover coefficient when 2SLS is employed (see Table A.2) reflects the correction for the negative effects of unionism on turnover.

TABLE A.3

Partial Results of Turnover Model
(dependent variable: turnover rate in the ith occupation)

Independent Variables	OLS	2SLS
Constant	.3179[a]	.0393
	(.0566)	(.1299)
Union membership	.01907	.1216
	(.0165)	(.07299)
Wage	.0123	.3854[a]
	(.0165)	(.1367)
N	601	495
$\overline{R}^2$	.054	—[b]

[a]Significant at .01 level.
[b]$\overline{R}^2$ not available for 2SLS.
Notes: The union measure is a continuous predicted value and should be evaluated at 1.00 and 0.0 for results similar to OLS. The wage variable is interpreted as discussed in the previous footnote.
The standard error of the regression coefficient is in parentheses.
Source: Compiled by the authors from mailed questionnaire.

The results in Table A.3 indicate unionism does, in fact, tend to reduce turnover and suggest an effect that is both statistically and "practically" significant. According to these results, occupations that are unionized experience a 12 percentage point decrease in annual turnover. Given a mean turnover rate of 23 percent for this group, it is clear that union effect is quite impressive. In addition, because the unionism variable is a predicted value and subject to measurement error as we discussed earlier, it probably represents a conservative estimate.

The effect of wages on turnover in the 2SLS results is positive as we suggested earlier in this section. The relationship is quite stable and probably reflects the higher turnover rates among those with clerical skills. The coefficient indicates that the $.20 per hour difference in wages among those with clerical skills and other workers is associated with nearly a 3 percentage point difference in annual turnover.

In sum, while these estimates are somewhat tentative, they point out the need to consider the potential simultaneity involved in the influence of collective bargaining on an organization. Based on these and additional three-stage least squares results, the interaction of collective bargaining, wages, and turnover in the hospital industry appears to operate in the following manner (at least among service workers).

High turnover, low wage workers, while traditionally not a target for organizing drives, are being successfully unionized because their demand for union services exceeds any reluctance on the part of the union to supply those services. The low wages reflect desires for economic gain, while high turnover rates characterize unsatisfactory working conditions. The union's willingness to work with these groups is in part due to a "social justice" interest, as well as a feeling that once organized, these workers can be stabilized and, therefore, not represent an undue expense to maintain the membership.

Finally, the union effects on wages are observed in two ways. First, we have the traditional union member coefficient, which in this sample is quite small and of little practical significance. However, more importantly, because turnover is negatively related to wages and unionization has been shown to reduce turnover by more than 50 percent in this sample, union members enjoy higher average wages because their turnover is reduced. The net result of these two effects is probably an 8 to 9 percent union/nonunion differential. While the magnitude of this estimate is not much different from that available through OLS, by using an improved estimation technique, we can see that the source of the union influence on wages is primarily derived from its stabilizing effect on its members.

NOTE

1. For a much more thorough discussion of this issue and the results, see Brian Becker, "The Impact of Unions on Labor Costs in Hospitals: A Three State Study" (Ph.D. diss.: University of Wisconsin, 1977).

BIBLIOGRAPHY

This bibliography covers material that examines the impact of collective bargaining on the administration of institutions in the health services industry. The focus is the issues involved, whether they be reported in a national sense or in the three states that came under scrutiny in the project. The time frame for the examination of the professional literature was basically the 1970s, through the beginning of 1979, though a smaller number of citations to signal articles and publications from the 1960s is also included.

The sources utilized for locating the bibliographical citations are listed below. Since no newspaper citations were included the interested reader should also consult the New York Times Index, the Wall Street Journal Index, and the indexes to such newspapers as the Los Angeles Times, the Washington Post, the Chicago Tribune, and the San Francisco Chronicle.

MEDICAL INDEXES

Abstracts of Hospital Management Studies
Cumulative Index to Nursing Literature
Excerpta Medica (Management Series)
Hospital Literature Index (formerly, Cumulative Index
    of Hospital Literature)
Index Medicus
International Nursing Index
Medical Care Review
Medical Socioeconomic Research Sources

OTHER INDEXES

Alternative Press Index
Business Periodicals Index
Cornell University Industrial Relations Library Catalog
Dissertations Abstracts
Index to U.S. Government Periodicals
Personnel Literature
Public Affairs Information Service Bulletin

<u>U.S. Department of Labor Library Catalog</u>
<u>Work-Related Abstracts</u> (formerly, <u>Employment</u>
<u>Relations Abstracts</u>)

The bibliography is arranged in the following categories. If
the subject matter seemed to call for it, an entry was made for a
work in more than one category.

BIBLIOGRAPHY CONTENTS

GENERAL CATEGORIES

Abelow, William J. "Labor Forecast: More Unions, More Government Control." Modern Hospital 119 (November 1972): 64-65.

Austin, M. J., et al. "Occupational Mental Health and the Human
Services: A Review." Health Social Work 2 (February 1977):
91-118.

Bailey, W. "Hospitals and Unions." Public Relations Journal 25
(February 1969): 6-9.

Bice, Michael O. "Building a Data Base." Hospitals 48 (June 16,
1974): 77-80.

Carlson, D. R. "Labor Union: Color It White, Black or Red."
Modern Hospital 105 (August 1965): 107-11.

"Charleston Blues." Economist 231 (May 3, 1969): 47-48.

"Charleston's Surrender." Economist 232 (July 12, 1969): 48.

Cleland, Virginia S. "To End Sex Discrimination." Nursing Clinics
of North America 9 (September 1974): 563-71.

"Costs, Unions, Regulations Dominate American Health Congress."
Hospital Medical Staff 3 (October 1974): 36-47.

Feinbaum, Robert. "Doctor and Public: An Appraisal of Professional Politics." Ph.D. dissertation, University of California
at Berkeley, 1967.

Ferguson, M. "The Dilemma of Professionalism and Nursing Organization." Nurse Mirror 143 (December 16, 1976): 61-64.

Gershenfeld, Walter. "Hospitals." In Emerging Sectors of Collective Bargaining, edited by Seymour Wolfbein, pp. 173-218.
Morristown, N.J.: General Learning Press, 1970.

Goldstein, Harold M. "More on Profits and Hospitals." Journal
of Economic Issues 5 (December 1971): 113-22.

Harris, Seymour E. The Economics of Health Care. Berkeley:
McCutchan, 1974.

Helin, E. B. "Hospitals: Over 40 or 8 and 80?" Personnel Journal 51 (August 1972): 565-70.

Hopping, B. "Professionalism and Unionism: Conflicting Ideologies." Nursing Forum 15 (1976): 372-83.

"Hospitals Face the Knife." Business Week, September 6, 1976, pp. 68-69.

"Hospital Organized Assigned to South." Retail, Wholesale and Department Stores Union Record 24 (May 1977): 7.

Kelly, Dorothy N. "Eagles Are Gathering—Again!" Supervisor Nurse 5 (October 1974): 6.

_____. "Right On—Into the Fray." Supervisor Nurse 5 (January 1974): 7.

Klarman, Herbert E. "Major Public Initiatives in Health Care." The Public Interest 34 (Winter 1974): 106-23.

Lewis, H. L. "Nurses: How Much Like Doctors?" Modern Health Care 3 (June 1975): 45-49.

Lihach, Nadine. "San Francisco: Winners and Losers." Modern Health Care, Short-Term Care Edition 2 (October 1974): 32-34.

"Local 1199 Urged to Put the Patient before the Union." Modern Hospital 119 (July 1972): 45.

Loveless, J. "ANA Labor Relations Workshops Win Encore." American Nurse 7 (May 1975): 6.

Miller, R. L. "Collective Bargaining: A New Frontier for Hospitals." Hospital Progress 56 (February 1975): 58.

Mitchell, Keith. "The Role of Labor." National Hospital 14 (September 1970): 29-34.

Nash, Al. "Hospital's Value System and the Union." Hospital Administration 19 (Fall 1974): 49-64.

"OR Nurse—Between Union and Management." Hospitals 48 (May 1, 1974): 77-81.

O'Rourke, K. D. "Christian Responsibility for Labor and Management." Hospital Progress 56 (July 1975): 62–66.

Phillips, Donald F. "New Demands on Nurses." Hospitals 48 (August 16, 1974): 31–34, and (September 16, 1974): 41–44.

Robbins, Anthony. "Professionalism and the Power of Management in Health Services." In Proceedings of the Twenty-Third Annual Winter Meeting of the Industrial Relations Research Association, edited by Gerald G. Somers, pp. 146–52. Madison: Industrial Relations Research Association, 1971.

Schorr, Thelma M. "They'd Better Believe." American Journal of Nursing 74 (August 1974): 1415.

Spiro, H. R., I. Siassi, and G. Crocetti. "Cost-Financial Mental Health Facility: III. Economic Issues and Implications for Future Patterns of Health Care." Journal of Nervous and Mental Disease 160 (April 1975): 249–54.

"Unions in Hospitals." Southern Hospitals 41 (March 1973): 4.

Weinmann, Richard A. "Unions: What Choice?" Cornell Hotel and Restaurant Administration 14 (August 1973): 13–15.

"William J. Usery, Jr., An interview with the director of the Federal Mediation and Conciliation Service." Hospitals 48 (September 16, 1974): 45–48.

Wurf, Jerry. "Union Clout in Health Care Reform." New Physician 20 (May 1971): 318–21.

"Your Opinion Please." Michigan Medicine 71 (November 1972): 956–58.

LABOR MARKET

General

Andrews, Theodora. A Bibliography of the Socioeconomic Aspects of Medicine. Littleton, Colo.: Libraries Unlimited, 1975.

Bishop, C. E. "Hospitals: From Secondary to Primary Labor Market." Industrial Relations 16 (July 1977): 26–34.

Breu, Theodore M. "Geographical and Professional Characteristics of Illinois Health Manpower—Distributional Factors and Determinants." Ph.D. dissertation, Southern Illinois University, 1972.

Brown, C. A. "Women Workers in the Health Service Industry." International Journal of Health Services 5 (1975): 173-84.

Kellam, Paul W. "A New Plan to Give Doctors Muscle with Government." Medical Economics 49 (February 14, 1972): 235-41.

Korst, Donald R. "Manpower Specialty in Wisconsin." Wisconsin Medical Journal 72 (April 1973): 107-12.

McNulty, M. F., Jr. "Health Manpower." Hospitals 40 (April 1, 1966): 83-88.

Medical Socioeconomic Research Sources. Chicago: American Medical Association, 1971.

Medical Socioeconomic Research Sources. Chicago: American Medical Association, 1972.

Metzger, Norman. "Training, Employment, Wages Soar as Health Care Industry Expands." Hospitals 50 (October 16, 1976): 67-70.

"The Hospitals and Health Manpower." Hospitals 39 (September 16, 1965): 94-96.

Supply and Demand

Adams, Frederick. "Manpower: A Real Issue in Urban Health." Urban Health 2 (August 1973): 8.

Bergen, Stanley S. "Physician Manpower: The Issues." Journal of the Medical Society of New Jersey 70 (August 1973): 557-60.

Bettis, Richard. "Survey Indicates Health Jobs Remain Unfilled." Texas Hospitals 29 (March 1974): 24.

Bognanno, Mario F., and Michael J. Delaney. "An Economic Analysis of the Future Work Plans of Inactive Married Professional Nurses." Industrial Relations Center, University of Minnesota, Reprint 93, 1973.

Bognanno, Mario F., J. S. Hixon, and J. R. Jeffers. "The Short-Run Supply of Nurse's Time." Industrial Relations Center, University of Minnesota, Reprint 92, 1974.

Bognanno, Mario F., James R. Jeffers, and Carol Oliven. "Evidence on the Physician Shortage." Industrial Relations Center, University of Minnesota, Reprint 94, 1971.

Bornmeier, Walter C. "Physician Shortage 1972." Journal of the American Medical Association 224 (May 14, 1973): 1033-34.

Cavert, H. Mead. "Projections of Future Need for Physicians in Minnesota." Minnesota Medicine 56 (June 1973): 529-33.

Cooper, James K., and Karen Heald. "Is There a Doctor Shortage?" Journal of the American Medical Association 227 (March 25, 1974): 1410-11.

Egeberg, R. O. "Allied Health Workers Now and Tomorrow." Manpower 2 (1970): 2-7.

Fischer, Donald. "The Physician Shortage: Some Solutions." Journal of the Arkansas Medical Society 70 (February 1974): 296.

Frey, Don C. "Manpower Realities and Health Care Costs." Paper presented at the University Consortium Conference for Comprehensive Health Planning, HEW Region III, May 30, 1974, in Pentagon City. (Available from American Association for Comprehensive Health Planning, Alexandria, Virginia.)

Ganong, W. L. "Shortage of Health Personnel: Crisis—or Chronic Situation?" Hospital Topics 44 (March 1966): 66-67.

Gerber, Alex. "Yes, There Is a Doctor Shortage." Prism 1 (August 1973): 13.

Greenfield, H. I., and C. A. Brown. Allied Health Manpower: Trends and Prospects. New York: Columbia University Press, 1969.

Hames, Myron Philip. "Laboratory Automation in Urban Hospitals: An Exploratory Study of the Effects of Automation on the Professional Role of Medical Technologists." Ph.D. dissertation, University of Florida, 1968.

Health Manpower—An Annotated Bibliography. Chicago: American
Hospital Association, 1972.

Hixon, Jesse S. "The Demand and Supply of Professional Hospital
Nurses: Intrahospital Resource Allocations." Ph.D. dissertation, Michigan State University, 1969.

Lewis, Charles E., M.D. "Health Manpower." Hospitals 46
(April 1, 1972): 107.

McConnell, John W. "Family Practitioners in Minnesota: Need and
Distribution." Minnesota Medicine 57 (April 1974): 319-22.

Miller, Winston, and Russell N. Hill. "Relationships between
Medical Education in Minnesota and Professional Location."
Minnesota Medicine 56 (April 1973): 329-32.

Millis, John S. "Diagnosing the Doctor Shortage." Nation's Business 62 (October 1964): 70-73.

Provost, George P. "Pharmacy Manpower: Numbers Game?"
American Journal of Hospital Pharmacy 30 (April 1973): 299.

Rayack, E. "Supply of Physician's Services." Industrial and Labor
Relations Review 17 (January 1964): 221-37.

Richardson, G. R. "Human Capital and the Market for Physicians
in the United States." Ph.D. dissertation, Columbia University,
1974.

Sloan, Frank A. "Physician Supply Behavior in the Short Run."
Industrial and Labor Relations Review 28 (July 1975): 549-69.

U.S., Department of Health, Education and Welfare. Manpower
Resources in Hospitals—1966: Summary Report of a Survey Con-
ducted by the Bureau of Health Manpower, Public Health Service,
Department of HEW and the American Hospital Association.
Chicago: American Hospital Association, 1967.

Weinstein, Bernard, and Doris Lesser. "Health Manpower."
Hospitals 48 (April 1, 1974): 67-72.

Yett, Donald E. An Economic Analysis of the Nurse Shortage.
Lexington, Mass.: Lexington, 1975.

Productivity, Costs, and Efficiency

Appelbaum, A. L. "New York City Hospitals: The Financial
Crunch." Hospitals 50 (January 16, 1976): 59-62.

Becker, Brian E. "The Impact of Unions on Labor Costs in Hospitals: A Three State Study." Ph.D. dissertation, University of
Wisconsin at Madison, 1977.

Carr, W. John, and Paul J. Feldstein. "The Relationship of Cost
to Hospital Size." Inquiry 4 (June 1967): 45-65.

Cohen, Harold A. "Variations in Cost among Hospitals of Different
Sizes." Southern Economic Journal 33 (January 1967): 355-58.

Collins, Gaum L. "Cost Analysis and Efficiency Measures for Hospitals." Inquiry 5 (June 1968): 50.

Ehrenberg, Ronald G. "Organizational Control and the Economic
Efficiency of Hospitals: The Production of Nursing Services."
The Journal of Human Resources 10 (Winter 1974): 21-32.

Feldstein, Martin S. Economic Analysis for Health Service Efficiency. Amsterdam: North Holland, 1967.

_____. "Hospital Cost Inflation: A Study of Nonprofit Price
Dynamics." American Economic Review 61 (December 1971):
853-72.

Fottler, Myron D. "The Effect of Workforce Skill Level and Work-
load on the Costs and Quality of Hospital Services." In Proceedings of the Twenty-Fourth Annual Winter Meeting of the Industrial
Relations Research Association, edited by Gerald G. Somers,
pp. 108-15. Madison: Industrial Relations Research Association,
1971.

McCormick, William, Jr. "Labor Relations and Labor Costs in
Hospitals." Ph.D. dissertation, Case Western Reserve University, 1968.

Spiro, H. R., I. Siassi, G. Crocetti, R. Ward, and E. Hanson.
"Cost-Financed Mental Health Facility: I. Clinical Care Pattern
in a Labor Union Program." Journal of Nervous and Mental
Disease 160 (April 1975): 249-54.

Spiro, H. R., I. Siassi, and G. Crocetti. "Cost-Financed Mental Health Facility: II. Utilization Profile of a Labor Union Program." Journal of Nervous and Mental Disease 160 (April 1975): 241-48.

Traska, M. R. "Hospitals Seek to Reduce Labor Cost." Modern Health Care 7 (August 1977): 50.

Turnover and Absenteeism

Adams, Jeffrey L. "The Costs and Benefits from Reducing Hospital Employee Turnover." Ph.D. dissertation, University of Pittsburgh, 1976.

Analyzing and Reducing Employee Turnover in Hospitals. New York: United Hospital Fund of New York, 1968.

Andy, E. "Hospital Turnover Problem." Personnel Administration (September-October 1965): 16-18.

Howell, D. L., and G. T. Stewart. "Labor Turnover in Hospitals." Personnel Journal 54 (December 1975): 624.

Kliesch, W. F., et al. "Absenteeism—A Study in Controls." Industrial Medicine and Surgery 35 (March 1966): 190-91.

Kliesch, W. F., and M. K. Wheeler. "A Hospital Health Service Evaluation of Absentee Control." Industrial Medicine and Surgery 38 (April 1969): 46-47.

Loungest, Beaufort B., Jr., and Donald E. Clawson. "The Effect of Selected Factors on Hospital Turnover Rates." Personnel Journal 53 (January 1974): 30-34.

Metzger, Norman. "Does Unionization of a Hospital Tend to Reduce Employee Turnover?" Hospital Personnel Administration Newsletter 8 (March 1972): 3.

Miner, M. G. "Job Absence and Turnover: A New Source of Data." Monthly Labor Review 100 (October 1977): 24-31.

Saleh, S. D. "Why Nurses Leave Their Jobs: An Analysis of Female Turnover." Personnel Administration 28 (January 1965): 25-28.

Snyder, S. M. "Controlling Absenteeism Can Help Curb Hospitals' Costs." Hospitals 52 (September 1, 1978): 102-3.

Strilaff, F. "Shiftwork and Turnover of General Duty Nurses." Dimensions of Health Service 53 (August 1976): 36-38.

Strossberg, Martin A. "The Impact of House Staff Turnover on Organizational Performance in Teaching Hospitals." Ph.D. dissertation, Syracuse University, 1977.

Tsui, A. "Diagnosis of Turnover Can Convert Causes to Assets." Hospitals 51 (July 16, 1977): 157-62.

Income Distribution and Wages

Brown, D. "Taft-Hartley Act: What Happens When It's Changed." Texas Nursing 48 (February 1974): 4-5.

Bryan, R. G. "Wages in Nursing Homes and Related Facilities." Monthly Labor Review 92 (May 1969): 61-62.

Bunker, Charles S. "Impact of Unionization on Wages of Nonmedical Hospital Employees." Hospital Topics 49 (January 1971): 31-32.

Bush, J. C. "Earnings of Hospital Employees." Monthly Labor Review 43 (October 1970): 90-91.

_____. "Nursing Home Wage Survey." Monthly Labor Review 98 (March 1975): 58-60.

"Earnings of Hospital Nurses." Monthly Labor Review 90 (June 1967): 55-58.

Fottler, Myron D. "Union Impact on Hospital Wages." Industrial and Labor Relations Review 30 (April 1977): 342-55.

Ginsburg, Helen. "Wage Differentials in Hospitals, 1956-1963: A Study Emphasizing the Wages of Nurses and Unskilled Workers in Nongovernment Hospitals." Ph.D. dissertation, New School for Social Research, 1967.

"Hospital Pact Brings Pay Hikes to 5000 Workers." Service Employee 36 (May 1977): 12.

"Hospital Wages Termed 'No Longer Substandard' at COLC Public Hearings in New York City." Hospitals 47 (November 16, 1973): 113.

King, Sandra L. "Wage Differences Narrow between Government and Private Hospitals." Monthly Labor Review 97 (April 1974): 56–57.

Lewis, L. E. "Earnings in Nursing Homes in April 1965." Monthly Labor Review 89 (March 1966): 291–95.

Salkever, David S. "Hospital Wage Inflation: Supply Push or Demand Pull?" Quarterly Review of Economics and Business 15 (Autumn 1975): 33–48.

Steele, Mark M. "Wages Rise Faster at Union Hospitals." Modern Health Care 6 (August 1976): 16–17.

Stelluto, G. L. "Earnings of Hospital Nurses, July 1966." Monthly Labor Review 90 (June 1967): 55–58.

Svettik, D. L., et al. "Job Clusters Studies Report More Accurate Wage–Salary Data." Hospitals 51 (August 1, 1977): 63–65.

U.S.; Department of Labor. Bureau of Labor Statistics. Hospitals, August 1972: Industry Wage Survey. Bulletin 1829. Washington, D.C.: Government Printing Office, 1974.

U.S., Department of Labor. Bureau of Labor Statistics. Industry Wage Survey: Nursing Homes and Related Facilities, May 1973. Bulletin 1855. Washington, D.C.: Government Printing Office, 1975.

U.S., Department of Labor. Bureau of Labor Statistics. Selected Earnings and Demographic Characteristics of Union Members, 1970. Report 417. Washington, D.C.: Government Printing Office, 1974.

U.S., Department of Labor. Office of Information. Bureau of Labor Statistics. Earnings and Supplementary Benefits in Hospitals—Chicago, Illinois. Washington, D.C.: Government Printing Office, 1973.

U.S., Department of Labor. Office of Information. Bureau of Labor Statistics. Earnings and Supplementary Benefits in Hospitals—Detroit, Michigan, August 1972. Washington, D.C.: Government Printing Office, 1973.

U.S., Department of Labor. Office of Information. Bureau of Labor Statistics. Earnings and Supplementary Benefits in Hospitals—Milwaukee, Wisconsin, August 1972. Washington, D.C.: Government Printing Office, 1973.

Manpower Programs

Bishop, Christene E. "Manpower Policy and the Supply of Nurses." Industrial Relations 12 (February 1973): 86-94.

Hahn, Jack A. L. "Development of New Kinds of Health Manpower." World Hospitals 10 (September 1974): 132-36.

Haskell, Mark A. The New Careers Concept: Potential for Public Employment of the Poor. New York: Praeger, 1969.

PERSONNEL MANAGEMENT

General

Ahmuty, A. L. "Legal and Personnel Problems of the Non-Union Hospitals." Virginia Nurse Quarterly 40 (Summer 1972): 17.

Alcade, J. J. "Hospital Unions: How to Deal with Them." Federation of American Hospitals Review 5 (October 1972): 40-41.

Alumkal, M. T. "A Survey of Personnel Policies and Practices in Metropolitan Chicago Hospitals." Ph.D. dissertation, University of Nebraska, 1967.

Bailey, Jack C. A Comparative Study of the Employment Conditions of Nurses (with and without Collective Bargaining). Washington, D.C.: George Washington University, 1965.

Basic Personnel Policies and Programs for a Health Care Institution: Guidelines for Development. Chicago: American Hospital Association, 1974.

Bates, D. L., and J. A. Wilterding. "How Unions Affect Hospital Administration." Health Services Manager 10 (November 1977): 7.

Bennett, Addison C. "Resisting Union Organizing Attempts." Hospital Topics 50 (January 1972): 30-34.

Bennett, Richard, and Ruth M. MacRobert. "Building Skills in Disciplining and Grievance Handling." Hospital Topics 53 (January-February 1975): 8, and 53 (March-April 1975): 50-55.

Benton, Douglas A. "Managerial Responsibilities for the Job Satisfaction of Registered Nurses." Ph.D. dissertation, Arizona State University, 1969.

Berkeley, A. Eliot, ed. Labor Relations in Hospitals and Health Care Facilities: Proceedings of a Conference Presented by the American Arbitration Association and the Federal Conciliation Service. Washington, D.C.: Bureau of National Affairs, 1976.

"Boards Cautioned re Labor Role." American Druggist 161 (June 29, 1970): 23.

Boyer, John M., et al. Employee Relations and Collective Bargaining in Health Care Facilities. St. Louis: C. V. Mosby, 1975.

Bulletin to Management no. 1202. Washington, D.C.: Bureau of National Affairs, 1973.

Cabot, Elaine E. "Know Your Employees or You Will Learn about Unions." Modern Hospital 119 (December 1972): 112.

Callan, Edward F. "Personnel Management in Hospitals." Hospital Topics 43 (December 1965): 27-28.

"Can Association's Good Offices Avert Pharmacy Unionism?" American Druggist Merchandising 168 (August 15, 1973): 61-62.

Centner, J. L. "Hospitals and Collective Bargaining." Personnel Journal 38 (November 1959): 203-5.

Cleland, Virginia S. "The Supervisor in Collective Bargaining." Journal of Nursing Administration 4 (1975): 33-35.

Clelland, Rod. The Human Side of Hospital Administration. Englewood Cliffs, N.J.: Prentice-Hall, 1974. Chapter 4.

Cokin, M. "Casework Principles Applied to Hospital Employment Problems." Personnel Journal 46 (March 1967): 170-73.

Colvecchio, R., B. Tescher, and C. Scalzi. "A Clinical Ladder for Nursing Practice." Journal of Nursing Administration 4 (1974): 54-58.

Connor, P. J. "Unions Are Here—Here's How to Cope." Modern Hospital 107 (August 1966): 102-4.

Dane, John Hunter. "A Model for Determining Turnover Costs." Hospitals 45 (May 16, 1972): 65-69.

Daykin, W. L. "Hospital Personnel Management in Transition." Personnel Administration 26 (September 1963): 37-41.

Dickenson, M. "Administrative Problems in Union Organizations." Royal Australian Nursing Federation Review 6 (May 1975): 7.

Doherty, V. C. "Emergence of Hospital Personnel Administration: An Exploratory Study of Hospitals in a Large Metropolitan Area." Dissertation Abstracts 28 (June 1968): 4795A. (Submitted to Michigan State University.)

"Do's and Don'ts for Management during Union Organization Drives." Hospital Food Service 4 (February 1971): 2-3.

"Economic, Political Woes Plague Public Hospitals: Sound, Hard-Headed Management Key to Solution." Hospitals 48 (January 1, 1974): 117-18.

Emanuel, William J. "Hospital Policy: Professional Associations as Unions." Hospital Progress 57 (January 16, 1976): 51-55.

Employee/Labor Relations Activity in Michigan Hospitals, December 31, 1973. Michigan Hospitals Association, Report no. 40. Washington, D.C., 1974.

Employee/Labor Relations Activity in Michigan Hospitals, June 30, 1974. Michigan Hospitals Association, Report no. 42. Washington, D.C., 1974.

Epstein, Richard L. "Employee Relations." Hospitals 49 (April 1, 1975): 75-77.

Falberg, Warren C. "Resisting Union Organizing Attempts." Hospital Topics 50 (January 1972): 30.

Foulkes, F. K. "The Expanding Role of the Personnel Function." Harvard Business Review 53 (March-April 1975): 71-84.

Ganong, Joan, and Warren Ganong. "Union Free Health Care Management?" Journal of Nursing Administration 3 (January-February 1973): 6.

Goldstein, Rhoda L., and Bernard Goldstein. Doctors and Nurses in Industry: Social Aspects of In-Plant Medical Programs. New Brunswick, N.J.: Rutgers University, Institute of Management and Labor, 1967.

Goodfellow, Matthew. "How the Union Organizer Rates Your Hospital: A Checklist." Administrative Briefs 7 (January 1973): 1-4.

_____. "How to Avoid Unionization." Hospital Housekeeping 3 (July-August 1974): 19-21.

_____. "Labor Unions: Are They Looking You Over?" Hospital World 2 (January 1973): 17-18.

Grand, K. N. "The Role of Ideology in the Unionization of Nurses." Abstracts of Hospital Management Studies 9. Cleveland: Case Western Reserve University, 1973.

Grant, R. A. "Cost Control under a Collective Agreement." Canadian Hospital 50 (April 1973): 10.

_____. "Impact of the Supervisor on the Collective Agreement." Canadian Hospital 49 (October 1972): 29.

Greenbaum, John S. "The Rebellious Rank and File." Personnel 49 (March-April 1972): 20-25.

Gregorich, Pauline, and James W. Long. "Responsive Management Fosters Cooperative Environment." Hospitals 50 (October 16, 1976): 99-104.

Gronbach, R. C. "Employee Participation as an Alternative to Unions." Hospital Topics 53 (September-October 1975): 27.

Hacker, R. L. "Organizational Systems for Change Offer an Alternative to Unions." Hospitals 50 (December 1, 1976): 45-47.

Haimann, Theo. Supervisory Management for Health Care Institutions. St. Louis: Catholic Hospital Association, 1973.

Hartnett, George D. A Comparative Survey of Selected Personnel
Activities between Those Acute General, Non-Profit Hospitals
and Those without Bargaining Units. Washington, D.C.: George
Washington University, School of Government, Business, and International Affairs, July 1969.

Hawkins, James L. "The Ward Manager System: A Case Study of
the Organization of Hospital Nursing Care." Ph.D. dissertation,
Purdue University, 1964.

"Health Care Bargaining: A Symposium." Employee Relations Law
Journal 1 (Winter 1976): 389-438.

Helin, E. B. "Hospitals: Over 40 or 8 and 80?" Personnel Journal
(August 1972): 565-70.

Hepner, James O., John M. Boyer, and Carl L. Westerhaus. Personnel Administration and Labor Relations in Health Care Facilities. St. Louis: C. V. Mosby, 1969.

Hilgert, Raymond L. "Why Your Employees Join a Union . . . An
Overview." Executive Housekeeper 18 (January 1972): 35.

Hoff, Wilbur. A Systems Approach to Health Manpower Utilization:
A Technical Procedures Manual. Oakland, Calif.: Institute for
Social Research, June 1, 1970 and May 31, 1973.

"Hospital Changes Advised to Deter Unionization." Hospitals 46
(April 16, 1972): 138.

"How to Win the Labor Tug of War." Modern Health Care, Short-
Term Care Edition 2 (September 1974): 56-60.

Hughes, L. E. "Industrial Services for the Nursing Home Industry."
Employment Service Review, August 1965, pp. 16-17.

Hunter, T. H. "Sounding Board. How Many Hats Can a House Officer Wear?" New England Journal of Medicine 294 (March 11,
1976): 608-9.

Imberman, A. A. "Are You the Type of Executive Who Causes Labor Trouble?" American Laundry Digest 37 (January 15, 1972): 70-74.

_____. "Communications: An Effective Weapon against Unionization." Hospital Progress 54 (December 1973): 54-57.

Jackson, L., et al. "Making Unions Unnecessary: The Supervisor and the New Employee." Journal of the American Health Care Association 3 (September 1977): 73-75.

_____. "Preventative Labor Relations—The Art of Making Unions Unnecessary." Journal of the American Health Care Association 2 (July 1976): 13-15.

_____. "Unions and the Facility: Why You Should Strive to Remain Free." Journal of the American Health Care Association 2 (May 1976): 15-17.

Jacox, Ada. The Nurse's Cap: A Case Study of Administrator Nurse Conflict. Cleveland: Case Western Reserve University, 1969.

James, Edward E. "If You Don't Listen to Employees' Complaints, Don't Be Surprised if a Union Does." Modern Nursing Home 28 (May 1972): 53-54.

_____. "Listen to Employees' Complaints and Then Do Something about Them." Modern Hospital 119 (July 1972): 61-62.

Jancura, Elise G. Labor Resource Utilization in Hospitals: Cost, Policies, and Recommendations. Cleveland: Bureau of Business Research, Cleveland State University, 1971.

_____. "The Economic Implications of the Use of Labor Resources by Hospitals." Ph.D. dissertation, Case Western Reserve University, 1971.

Johnson, Alton C. Human Resources Management, (Health Industry): Selected Bibliography. School of Business, University of Wisconsin at Madison (s.l. s.n. 1976): pp. 19-23.

Keaton, Harry J. "Hospitals Urged to Give Labor-Public Relations Top Priority." Public Relations Newsletter 19 (November 1970): 1-5.

Keefe, William F. "Seven Deadly Sins of Employee Relations."
American Laundry Digest 36 (March 15, 1971): 60.

Kinsella, C. R. "Administrative Reviews: Nursing." Hospitals 49
(April 1, 1975): 101-5.

Kludt, John W. "Tighter Operational Control Stimulated Union
Action." Hospital Management 99 (March 1965): 29-34.

Krinsky, Edward B. "Problems of Discipline and Discharge."
Hospitals 48 (May 16, 1974): 48-50.

"Labor and the Non-Profit Hospital: Are You Ready?" Personnel
Journal 53 (March 1974): 216.

LaMotte, Thomas. "Making Employee Orientation Work." Personnel Journal 53 (January 1974): 35.

Laner, Richard W. "Employer-Employee Relations: Unions and
Hospitals." Radiologic Technology 46 (July-August 1974): 10-19.

Levey, Samuel, and Paul N. Loomba. Health Care Administration:
A Managerial Perspective. Philadelphia: Lippincott, 1973.

Long, F., and D. Michelson. "Administrators: Don't Let Unions
Throw You for a Loss." Hospital Forum California 19 (April
1977): 10.

Lynn, N. B., et al. "Challenges of Men in a Women's World."
Public Personnel Management 40 (January 1975): 4-17.

Lyon, H. L., and J. M. Ivancevich. "Exploratory Investigation of
Organization Climate and Job Satisfaction in a Hospital." Academy of Management Journal 17 (December 1974): 635-48.

MacBain, N. "Administrative Reviews: Volunteer Services."
Hospitals 49 (April 1, 1975): 117.

"Managing Industrial Action." Hospital and Health Services Review
70 (February 1974): 41.

Martin, J. C. "Planning for Summer Staff Shortages." Dimensions
of Health Service 55 (July 1978): 10-11.

Match, Robert K., et al. "Unionization, Strikes, Threatened Strikes and Hospitals—The View from Hospital Management." International Journal of Health Services 5 (1975): 27–36.

McGhee, John R. "Lord, Why Me?" Osteopathic Hospital 18 (January 1974): 3–7.

Mecklin, J. M. "Hospitals Need Management Even More Than Money." Fortune 81 (January 1970): 96–99.

Metzger, Norman. "Is Union Organization of the Employees in Your Hospital Inevitable?" Hospital Management 112 (July 1971): 14–15.

_____. "The Role of the Supervisor in the Unionization of Employees." Hospital Management 112 (August 1971): 10.

_____. "The Six Forms of Union Security." Hospital Management 112 (September 1971): 11.

Meyer, G. D. "Determinants of Collective Action Attitudes among Hospital Nurses: An Empirical Test of a Behavioral Model." Ph.D. dissertation, University of Iowa, 1970.

Miller, Ronald L. "Anticipate Questions, Seek Answers for Adept Labor Relations Efforts." Hospitals 50 (July 1, 1976): 50–54.

_____. "Development and Structure of Collective Bargaining among Registered Nurses." Personnel Journal 50 (February–March 1971): 134.

Monium, George Francis. "Unionization and the Nursing Home Administrator." Journal of the American College of Nursing Home Administrators 2 (Summer 1974): 47–52.

Mote, John R. "Personnel Management." Hospitals 47 (April 1, 1973): 71.

Nash, Al. "Hospital Technology: Prescription for Peace?" Personnel Management 7 (1975): 24–27.

_____. "Hospital Values, Conflicts and Supervision Practices." Personnel Journal 52 (December 1973): 1056–60.

National Personnel Relations Committee of the American Society of Medical Technologists. Personnel Relations Handbook. Houston: American Society of Medical Technologists, 1970.

"Obligatory Triad: The Conflict in Hospital Administration." Personnel Journal 47 (August 1968): 582-84.

Olsson, D. E. "New Management Practices for the Small Organization." Advanced Management 26 (March 1961): 14-17.

Osterhaus, Leo B. "The Effect of Unions on Hospital Management." In Hospital Organization and Management, edited by Jonathan S. Rakich. St. Louis: Catholic Hospital Association, 1972, pp. 240-48.

_____. "The Industrial Relations System in the Hospital Industry." Personnel Journal 47 (May 1968): 315-20 and (June 1968): 412-19.

Packer, Clinton L. Preparing Hospital Management for Labor Contract Negotiations. Chicago: American Hospital Association, 1975.

"Physicians' Attitude Survey." Medical Opinion, July 1972, pp. 23-24.

Plachy, Roger J. "If You Lead, a Union Can't." Modern Health Care, Short-Term Edition 2 (November 1974): 116.

"Poll Shows Administrators Don't Want Unionization." Modern Nursing Home 28 (May 1972): 4.

Pomrinse, David S., M.D. "The Crisis in the Health Care System: A Contrary Opinion." Hospital Administration 19 (Winter 1974): 10-29.

Ponlin, M. "United States Government as Employer." Supervisor Nurse 3 (August 1972): 50-53.

Portelli, Andrew R. "Coordination of Personnel." Association of Operating Room Nurses Journal 16 (September 1972): 91-97.

"Preventing Unionization." Hospital Food Service 7 (August 1974): 2-3.

Quay, Charles. "Watch Out! Here Come the Unions." Food Management 8 (July 1973): 50-51.

Rakich, Jonathan S., ed. Hospital Organization and Management: A Book of Readings. St. Louis: Catholic Hospital Association, 1972.

Rakich, Jonathan S. "Hospital Unionization Causes and Effects." Hospital Administration 18 (Winter 1973): 7-18.

_____. "Personnel Practices in Long-Term Care Facilities." Hospital Progress 55 (May 1974): 64.

Reinhold, C. Ross. "Some Aspects of Motivation of Hospital Workers." Master's thesis, University of Wisconsin at Madison, 1969.

Rombach, M. E. "A Hospital's Commitment to Just and Equitable Personnel Policies." Hospital Progress 56 (July 1975): 57.

Rothman, William A. "Administrative Problems in the Hospital." Michigan Hospitals 7 (October 1971): 8-11.

Ruchlin, Hirsch S., et al. "Health Administration Manpower Research: A Critique and a Proposal." Hospital Administration 18 (Summer 1973): 81-103.

Samaras, J. T. "Administrative Attitudes on Collective Bargaining in Hospitals." Supervisor Nurse 9 (January 1978): 56.

Sampson, Arthur J. "Labor Unions and the Nursing Home." Journal of the American College of Nursing Home Administrators 2 (Summer 1974): 37-46.

Schulz, Rockwell, and Alton C. Johnson. Management of Hospitals. New York: McGraw-Hill, 1976. Chapter 14.

Shaw, David G. Meeting Health Manpower Needs through More Effective Use of Allied Health Workers. U.S. Department of Labor Manpower Research Monograph, no. 25. Washington, D.C.: Government Printing Office, 1973.

Silver, D. F. "Counseling and Peer Review Are Key Disciplinary Procedures." Hospitals 52 (August 1, 1978): 189-90.

"Six-Point Program to Implement Now before Unionization Drives Begin." Hospital Financial Management 4 (November 1974): 23.

Sloan, Stanley, and David E. Schrieber. Hospital Management. Madison: University of Wisconsin, Graduate School of Business, Bureau of Business Research and Service, 1971.

Smejda, Hellena. "Unions Are Coming Your Way." Hospital Financial Management 4 (November 1974): 12.

Sorenson, B. D. "Emphasizing Personnel-Employer Relationships in Texas Hospitals." Texas Hospitals 30 (September 1974): 4-5.

Spencer, Vernon. "The Nurse and Her Employee Labor Relations Say Unions Are Here to Stay." Hospital Management 97 (April 1964): 49-51.

_____. "The Nurse and Her Employee Labor Relations, Part 2. The Problems That Arise Most Frequently between Nurses and the Union." Hospital Management 97 (May 1974): 44-48.

Stanton, Erwin S. "White Collar Unionization: New Challenge to Management." Personnel Journal 51 (February 1972): 118-24.

Steve, Laurence. "Labor Negotiations and the Director of Physical Therapy." Physical Therapy 53 (June 1973): 623-27.

Stevens, B. J. "The Problem in Nursing's Middle Management." Journal of Nursing Administration 4 (1974): 37-40.

Sweeney, Sister Margaret, and Edith H. Belsjoe. "Employee Communications during and after a Union Campaign." Hospital Progress 55 (April 1974): 52.

Tappan, Francis Marie. "Toward Understanding Hospital Administration." Ph.D. dissertation, Columbia University, 1967.

Ten Boer, Marlin H. "Study of the Extent and Impact of Organized Labor in Colleges and Universities." Ed.D. dissertation, Indiana University, 1970. Also in Journal of the College and University Personnel Association 22 (December 1970): 27-73.

Torrence, William D. "Educating and Training Management in Collective Bargaining and Labor Relations." Hospital Progress 54 (May 1973): 78-83.

_____. "Health Services and Collective Bargaining: An Approach to Management Education and Training." Training Development Journal 28 (August 1974): 36-39.

"Union Benefits Questioned." American Medical News 15 (May 29, 1972): 1.

Wagner, E. "Avoiding Illegal Employment Practices." Hospitals
49 (June 16, 1975): 45-49.

Wallace, M. J., et al. "Measurement Modifications for Assessing
Organizational Climate in Hospitals." Academy of Management
Journal 18 (March 18, 1975): 82-97.

Williard, William R. "How Health Manpower Problems Affect the
System." Hospital Medical Staff 3 (May 1974): 1-9.

Wollenberger, Joseph B. "Honesty Is the Key to Coexistence with
Unions." Modern Hospital 114 (February 1970): 102-3.

Wren, George R. "Personnel Administration in Hospitals." Personnel Journal 52 (January 1973): 54-56.

Selection and Training

Abernathy, W. J. "Nursing Staffing Problems: Issues and Prospects." Sloan Management Review 13 (Fall 1971): 87-99.

Alcade, J. J. "Hospital Unions: How to Deal with Them." Federation of American Hospitals Review 5 (October 1972): 40-41.

Fiester, K. "Upgrading Hospital Workers." Manpower 2 (August
1970): 24-27.

Fottler, Myron D. "Administrative View of Manpower Utilization
in the Hospital." Personnel Journal (July 1972): 505-10.

_____. "Manpower Substitution in the Hospital Industry: An Ex-
ploratory Study of the New York City Voluntary and Municipal
Hospital System." Ph.D. dissertation, Columbia University, 1970.

Goldstein, Harold M., Morris A. Horowitz, and Kathleen A. Calore.
Improving the Utilization of Health Manpower. Boston: Northeastern University, Department of Economics, Center for Medical Manpower Studies, 1974.

"Hospital Now Teaching Personnel Development." Personnel 46
(1969): 7.

"Joint Hospital-Union Training at Mount Sinai." Training and Development Journal 21 (January 1967): 46.

Torrence, William D. "Health Services and Collective Bargaining: An Approach to Management Education and Training." Training Development Journal 28 (August 1974): 36-39.

Compensation Policies

Beissel, J. J. "Recognition of Professional Preparation: The Key to Job Evaluation in Health Care Facilities." Personnel Journal 51 (February 1972): 136-37.

Bristow, Charles S. "A Description and Exploratory Analysis of Unionization and Its Effect on Costs, Employee Compensation and Compensation Programs in the Voluntary Not-for-Profit Hospital." Master's thesis, University of Alabama, 1972.

"Cost of Living Payments as an Aid to Wage and Salary Stability." Personnel Journal 48 (1969): 655-56.

Crosley, W. D. "Progressive Wage and Salary Programming in the Hospital." Personnel Journal 49 (August 1970): 655-61.

Daniels, Charles. What Is Adequate Employee Compensation?" Michigan Hospitals 10 (May 1974): 6-9.

"Financial Incentives Invalidate Union Election." Newsletter of the American Society of Hospital Attorneys 6 (March 1973): 3-4.

Franklin, Stephen. Fringe Benefits, Hospitals, and Unions. Iowa City: University of Iowa, 1968. (University Microfilms #298.)

Jehring, J. J. "A Planning Guide: Designing Systems Incentive Programs for Hospital Employees." Madison: University of Wisconsin, Center for the Study of Productivity Motivation, 1969.

Leathem, R. M. "Wage and Salary Administration in Hospitals." Canadian Hospital 43 (March 1966): 46-49.

Petersen, D. J. "Labor Trends: White Collar Unionization and the Pay Board." Personnel 49 (July-August 1972): 34-39.

LABOR LAW

General

Abelow, William J. "Labor Forecast: More Unions, More Government Control." Modern Hospital 119 (November 1972): 64-65.

Ahmuty, A. L. "Legal and Personnel Problems of the Non-Union Hospital." Virginia Nurse Quarterly 40 (Summer 1972): 17.

Amundson, Norman E. "Labor Relations and the Nursing Leader (Labor Laws)." Journal of Nursing Administration 4 (September-October 1974): 10-12.

_____. "The Rules of the Game Are Changing." Journal of Nursing Administration 1 (May-June 1971): 45-49.

Anderson, Betty Jane. "Unions—The Legal Aspects." Connecticut Medicine 37 (April 1973): 212-13.

Bader, Albert X., Jr. "Collective Bargaining in Hospitals and Other Nonprofit Operations." In Proceedings of New York University Nineteenth Annual Conference on Labor, pp. 235-63. Washington, D.C.: Bureau of National Affairs, 1967.

Baird, N. M. "Barriers to Collective Bargaining in Registered Nursing." Labor Law Journal 20 (January 1969): 42-46.

Ballenger, Martha D. "A New Approach to the Legal Regulation of Health Personnel." In Proceedings of the Twenty-Third Annual Winter Meeting of the Industrial Relations Research Association, edited by Gerald G. Somers. Madison: Industrial Relations Research Association, 1971.

Barnes, David L. "Collective Bargaining for Radiologic Technologists." Radiologic Technology 45 (September-October 1973): 79-88.

Barrett, Jerome T., and Ira B. Lobel. "Public Sector Strikes—Legislative and Court Treatment." Monthly Labor Review 97 (September 1974): 19-22.

Bernstein, Arthur H. "Law in Brief (Hospitals and Labor Laws)." Hospitals 47 (December 1, 1973): 110-12.

Bornstein, Timothy, ed. Health Care Labor Manual. 3 vols. Rockville: Skoler and Abbott, 1974.

Bottone, Anthony. "Physicians and Labor Laws." The New Physician 21 (December 1972): 739-40.

"Chaotic Controls: Unions Grab, Hospitals Grope." Hospital World 1 (February 1972): 1.

Clark, James R. A Study of Labor Law and Relations in Carolina Hospitals. Durham, N.C.: Duke University, 1974.

Craver, C. B. "The Application of Labor and Antitrust Laws to Physician Unions: The Need for a Re-evaluation of Traditional Concepts in a Radically Changing Field." Hastings Law Journal 2 (September 1975): 55-97.

Creighton, H. "Law for the Nurse-Supervisor." Supervisor Nurse 3 (March 1972): 8.

Crouch, Winston W. "Local Government Labor Relations Today." Public Management 57 (February 1975): 4-6.

Cunningham, Robert M. "Looking Around: That's Not What They Had in Mind." Modern Health Care 4 (August 1975): 10-16.

Ecenbarger, William. "Second Thoughts about the Right to Strike." Private Practice 5 (July 1973): 36-37.

Eisner, Eugene G., and Phillip Sipser. "Charleston Hospital Dispute: Organizing Public Employees and the Right to Strike." St. John's Law Review 45 (December 1970): 254-72.

The Federal Mediation and Conciliation Service and Its Role in the Health Care Industry: A Handbook. Washington, D.C.: Federal Mediation and Conciliation Service, n.d.

Francke, Don E. "Meeting the Challenge of Change." American Journal of Hospital Pharmacy 27 (March 1970): 188-99.

Gamm, Sara. Toward Collective Bargaining in Non-Profit Hospitals: Impact of New York Law. New York State School of Industrial and Labor Relations Bulletin no. 60. Ithaca, N.Y.: Cornell University, 1968.

Gordon, Murray A. "Hospital Housestaff Collective Bargaining." Employee Relations Law Journal 1 (Winter 1976): 418-38.

Gowing, Robert E. The Timing of Management Decisions during a Union Organization Attempt. Birmingham: University of Alabama, 1976. Available from Xerox University Microfilms (reel 1165).

"Health Care Bargaining: A Symposium." Employee Relations Law Journal 1 (Winter 1976): 389-438.

Holloway, Sally T. "Health Professionals and Collective Action." Employee Relations Law Journal 1 (Winter 1976): 410-17.

Kleingartner, Archie. "Nurses, Collective Bargaining and Labor Legislation." Labor Law Journal 18 (April 1967): 236-45.

"Labor Issues Affecting Health Care Institutions." Labor Relations Reporter, Background News and Information, May 26, 1975, pp. 89LRR80-89LRR83.

Loveless, J. "Interns, Residents Change Bylaws; Begin Aggressive Organizing Efforts." American Nurse 7 (November 28, 1975): 7.

Meltzer, Bernard D. "The Doctors' Right to Strike." Labor Law Journal (February 1963): 216-19.

"More Not Less, Federal Regulation Predicted for Health Care Field." Hospitals 48 (June 1, 1974): 122-24.

Munger, Mary D. "Nursing Supervision and Labor Laws." Supervisor Nurse 3 (September 1972): 15.

"New Executive Order Governs Federal Agency Bargaining." American Journal of Nursing 70 (January 1970): 13.

"Plight of Non-Profit Hospital Employees." Laborer 27 (November 1973): 8-9.

Schmidman, J. "Nurses and Pennsylvania's New Public Employee Bargaining Law." Labor Law Journal 22 (November 1971): 725-33.

Somers, Anne R. Hospital Regulation: The Dilemma of Public Policy. Princeton: Princeton University, Industrial Relations Section, 1969.

"Special Report on Physicians' Unions: What Are They . . . Recent Developments . . . Legal Aspects." Delaware Medical Journal 45 (February 1973): 44-48.

"Speakers Tell ACHA That Issues Are Consumerism, Government Control, and Housestaff-Hospital Relations." Modern Hospital 120 (March 1973): 47.

Sweeney, Sister Margaret, and Edith H. Belsjoe. "Employee Communications during and after a Union Campaign." Hospital Progress 55 (April 1974): 52.

Wagner, E. "Avoiding Illegal Employment Practices." Hospitals 49 (June 16, 1975): 45-49.

Pre-1974 Taft-Hartley Amendments

Bernstein, Arthur H. "Hospitals and Labor Laws." Hospitals 47 (December 1, 1973): 110-12.

Emanuel, William J. "Nonprofit Hospitals and the NLRA Exemption." Hospital Progress 54 (January 1973): 69.

_____. "Taft-Hartley Exemption." Hospitals 45 (April 16, 1971): 66-68.

"Exemption of Nonprofit Hospital Employees from the National Labor Relations Act: A Violation of Equal Protection." Iowa Law Review 57 (December 1971): 412-50.

Hoover, Earl R. "At Common Law—the Hospital." Labor Law Journal 18 (August 1967): 460-67.

"Hospitals Need Special Labor Laws, New Yorker Asserts." Modern Hospital 116 (April 1971): 34.

"Hospitals Criticized for Fighting to Maintain Exemption from Labor Management Laws." Hospitals 44 (November 16, 1970): 114.

"Labor Law: Hospital Employees." University of Illinois Law Forum 3 (1973): 542-62.

March, David C. "Industrial Relations Act Code of Practice." Hospital and Health Services Review 68 (December 1972): 440-43.

Olson, Donald R. "Breaking Trail in the NLRB: A Case Study Report." Medical Group Management 20 (September–October 1973): 14-17.

"Pharmacy Intern Is Not a Professional, at Least as far as Union Bargaining Is Concerned Says NLRB." American Druggist 154 (August 1, 1966): 20.

Pointer, Dennis D. "Federal Labor Law Status of the Health Care Delivery Industry." Labor Law Journal 22 (May 1971): 278-86.

_____. "Hospital Labor Relations Legislation: An Examination and Critique of Public Policy." Hospital Progress 54 (January 1973): 71-75.

_____. "Labor Law Status of Health Care Facilities." Hospital Progress 51 (September 1970): 44-47, (October 1970): 83-86, and (November 1970): 72-75.

_____. "Prospects for Removing the Taft-Hartley Exemption." Hospital Progress 55 (March 1974): 43-45.

_____. "Toward a National Hospital Labor Relations Policy: An Examination of Legislative Exemption." Labor Law Journal 23 (April 1972): 238-48.

"Private Physician Unions: Federal Antitrust and Labor Law Implications." UCLA Law Review 20 (June 1973): 983-1014.

Rayburn, John Michael. "Barriers to Collective Bargaining in the Profession of Pharmacy." Hospital Pharmacy 5 (November 1970): 11-14.

Soderholm, John C. Guidelines for the Design of Voluntary Nonprofit Hospital Labor Legislation. St. Louis: Washington University School of Medicine, Graduate Program in Health Care Administration, June 1971.

Somers, Anne R. Hospital Regulation: The Dilemma of Public Policy. Princeton: Princeton University, Industrial Relations Section, 1969.

U.S., Department of Labor. National Labor Relations Board. Quarterly Report of the General Counsel. Washington, D.C.: Government Printing Office, 1973.

"Unions May Enforce Employee's Rights against Not-for-Profit Hospitals." Newsletter of the American Society of Hospital Attorneys 6 (November 1973): 5.

Weissbrodt, Sylvia. "Changes in State Labor Laws in 1972." Monthly Labor Review 96 (January 1973): 27-36.

Post-1974 Taft-Hartley Amendments

Cleland, Virginia. "Taft-Hartley Amended: Implications for Nursing—The Professional Model." American Journal of Nursing 75 (February 1975): 288-92.

Despres, L. M. "What the National Labor Relations Act Really Says." American Journal of Nursing 76 (May 1976): 790-94.

"Doctors Hit the Streets with a New Strike Law." Business Week, March 31, 1975, pp. 19-20.

Emanuel, William J. "Coping with the NLRA." Hospital Forum (California) 17 (November 1974): 15-16.

"Employees in Community Hospitals Given Green Light to Organize." Medical World News 15 (August 9, 1974): 66-68.

Epstein, Richard L. "The Legal Perspective." Trustee 288 (January 1975): 17-19.

Etheridge, Lucille L. "Cornering Current Concerns." Journal of Practical Nursing 23 (October 1974): 15.

"Extension of Taft-Hartley Act to Nonprofit Hospitals Discussed by Nash." White Collar Report 898 (June 14, 1974): A14-15.

Farkas, Emil C. "The National Labor Relations Act: The Health Care Amendments." Labor Law Journal 25 (May 1978): 259-74.

Feheley, Lawrence F. "Amendments to the National Labor Relations Act: Health Care Institutions." Ohio State Law Journal 36 (1975): 235-98.

Friedman, Edward D. "Newington Children's Hospital." American Occupational Therapy Association amicus curiae brief filed before the NLRB, January 27, 1975.

Graham, Harry E. "Effects of NLRB Jurisdictional Change on Union Organizing Activity in the Proprietary Health Care Sector." In Proceedings of the Twenty-Fourth Annual Winter Meeting of the Industrial Relations Research Association, edited by Gerald G. Somers. Madison: Industrial Relations Research Association, 1971.

"Guidelines of National Labor Relations Board General Counsel on Handling ULP Cases under Nonprofit Hospital Amendments." White Collar Report 908 (August 23, 1974): C1-14.

"Health Care Bargainings: A Symposium." Employee Relations Law Journal 1 (Winter 1976): 389-438.

Hollendorfer, C. A. "Your Rights under NLRB." Colorado Nurse 75 (February 1975): 7.

Holloway, Sally T. "Health Professionals and Collective Action." Employee Relations Law Journal 1 (Winter 1976): 410-17.

"Hospital and Nursing Discipline: Nurses' Rights . . . Unfair Labor Practice Complaints." Regan Report on Nursing Law 18 (September 1977): 2.

Kane, T. J. "Non-Profit Hospitals and the National Labor Relations Act—First Issues." Journal of Nursing Administration 5 (July-August 1975): 15.

Katz, Barbara F. "Nonprofit Hospital Amendment to the National Labor Relations Act." Medicological News 3 (January 1975): 1.

Leininger, M. "Taft-Hartley Amended: Implications for Nursing—Conflict and Conflict Resolution." American Journal of Nursing 75 (February 1975): 284-88.

Lewis, Howard L. "Wave of Union Organizing Will Follow Break in the Taft-Hartley Dam." Modern Health Care, Short-Term Edition 1 (May 1974): 25-32.

Loveless, J. "Interns, Residents Change Bylaws: Begin Aggressive Organizing Effort." American Nurse 7 (November 28, 1975): 7.

_____. "NLRB Rules on Nursing's Community of Interest." American Nurse 7 (June 1975): 1.

Metzger, Norman. "NLRA Boards of Inquiry Have Been Used Sparingly." Hospitals 50 (July 1, 1976): 55-57.

Munger, Mary D. "Labor Relations Act: Implications for Nurses." Association of Operating Room Nurses Journal 19 (May 1974): 1127-32.

National Labor Relations Board. General Counsel, Memorandum. Guidelines for Handling Unfair Labor Practice Cases Arising under the 1974 Nonprofit Hospital Amendments to the Act. Washington, D.C.: National Labor Relations Board, August 20, 1974.

"National Labor Relations Board Criteria for Determining the Status of Charge Nurses." Hospitals 50 (June 1, 1976): 45.

"National Labor Relations Board Issues Hospital Union Rules." American Medical News 18 (May 1975): 1.

Phillips, Donald F. "Taft-Hartley: What to Expect." Trustee 27 (December 1974): 23-28.

Pointer, Dennis D. "1974 Health Care Amendments to the National Labor Relations Act." Labor Law Journal 26 (June 1975): 350-59.

Pointer, Dennis D., and Norman Metzger. The National Labor Relations Act: A Guidebook for Health Care Facility Administrators. New York: Spectrum, 1975.

"Questions and Answers about Effects of Taft-Hartley Amendments." Colorado Nurse 76 (June 1976): 6.

Reimer, D. M. "The National Labor Relations Board—What It Does." American Association of Nurse Anesthetists Journal 43 (June 1975): 299-301.

Reimer, D. M., and M. M. Poulos. "National Labor Relations Board and Taft-Hartley Amendments, One Year Later." American Association of Nurse Anesthetists Journal 43 (December 1975): 618-25.

Rosmann, Joseph. "One Year under Taft-Hartley." Hospitals 49 (December 16, 1975): 64-68.

Shepard, Ira M. "Health Care Institution Amendments to the National Labor Relations Act: An Analysis." American Journal of Law and Medicine 1 (1975): 41-53.

"Statement of Illinois Nurses' Association on the Effect of the 1974 Taft-Hartley Amendments on Hospital Relationships with Nurses' Associations." Supervisor Nurse 6 (September 1975): 8-9.

"Taft-Hartley." Modern Health Care 2 (September 1974): 85.

The Status of Supervisors under the NLRA. Health/Labor Management Report, vol. 3. Mount Arlington, N.J.: Girard Associates, 1975.

U.S., Congress, House. Legislative History of H.R. 11357 to Amend the National Labor Relations Act to Extend Its Coverage and Protection to Employees of Nonprofit Hospitals. 93rd Cong., 2d sess. Washington, D.C.: Government Printing Office, 1973.

U.S., Congress, House. Committee on Education and Labor. Extension of NLRA to Nonprofit Hospital Employees: Hearings on H.R. 1236, a Bill to Amend the National Labor Relations Act to Extend Its Coverage to Employees of Nonprofit Hospitals. 93rd Cong., 2d sess. Washington, D.C.: Government Printing Office, 1973.

U.S., Congress, House. Committee on Education and Labor. Special Subcommittee on Labor. Extension of NLRA to Nonprofit Hospital Employees: Hearings on H.R. 11357 before Special Subcommittee on Labor. 92d Cong., 1st and 2d sess., 1971. Washington, D.C.: Government Printing Office, 1972.

U.S., Congress, Senate. Legislative History of S. 3203, to Amend the National Labor Relations Act to Extend Its Coverage and Protection to Employees of Nonprofit Hospitals. 93rd Cong., 2d sess. Approved July 26, 1974. Public Law 93-360. Washington, D.C.: Government Printing Office, 1974.

U.S., Congress, Senate. Legislative History of the Nonprofit Hospitals under the National Labor Relations Act, 1974. 93rd Cong., 2d sess. Washington, D.C.: Government Printing Office, 1974.

U.S., Congress, Senate. Committee on Education and Labor. Coverage of Nonprofit Hospitals under National Labor Relations Act, 1973. Hearings on S. 794 . . . and S. 2292 to Amend the National Labor Relations Act to Extend Its Coverage and Protection to Employees of Nonprofit Hospitals, and for Other Purposes. 93rd Cong., 1st sess. Washington, D.C.: Government Printing Office, 1973.

Wagner, E. "Avoiding Illegal Employment Practices." Hospitals 49 (June 16, 1975): 45-49.

"What Hospital Leaders Think about the Taft-Hartley Amendment." Hospital Progress 55 (September 1974): 26-27.

Zimmerman, A. "Taft-Hartley Amended: Implications for Nursing. The Industrial Model." American Journal of Nursing 75 (February 1975): 284-88.

Special Issues

Unit Determination

Abelow, William J. "Labor Forecast: More Unions, More Government Control." Modern Hospital 119 (November 1972): 64-65.

Alper, Philip R., ed. Doctors' Unions and Collective Bargaining. Report of a Proceedings Conference of the Institute of Industrial Relations and American Federation of Physicians and Dentists, at the University of California at Berkeley, 1974.

Baumgartner, R. P. "Hospital Pharmacy Is Seen Facing Wave of Unionism." American Druggist 170 (September 1, 1974): 64-66.

"Eighteen Hospital Groups Plan Powerful Bargaining Unit." American Druggist 166 (July 10, 1972): 28.

Emerson, W. L. "Appropriate Bargaining Units for Health Care Professional Employees." Journal of Nursing Administration 8 (September 1978): 10-15.

Jackson, L., et al. "No Solicitation, No Distribution." American Health Care Association Journal 2 (November 1976): 7-9.

Kruger, D. H. "Appropriate Bargaining Unit for Professional Nurses." Labor Law Journal 19 (January 1968): 3-11.

Loveless, J. "NLRB Rules on Nursing's Community of Interest." American Nurse 7 (June 1975): 1.

"National Labor Relations Board Gives General Approval to Separate Bargaining Units for Maintenance Employees in Hospitals." Hospitals 50 (May 1, 1976): 19-20.

Pepe, S. P. "Appropriate Health Care Bargaining Units: An Unsettled Question." Hospital Progress 58 (January 1977): 54.

Pepe, S. P., and R. L. Murphy. "The NLRB Decisions on Appropriate Bargaining Units." Hospital Progress 56 (August 1975):
43.

Solicitation

Barnes, David L. "Collective Bargaining for Radiologic Technologists: Organizational Vehicles." Radiologic Technology 46
(January-February 1975): 282-93.

Emanuel, William J., and Alfred Klein. "Solicitation Rules Will
Need Revision." Hospitals 49 (August 16, 1975): 47-51.

Epstein, R. L. "Guide to NLRB Rules on Solicitation and Distribution." Hospitals 49 (August 16, 1975): 43-47.

"Supreme Court Rules Hospitals Cannot Ban Union Activities in
Cafeteria and Coffee Shop." Hospitals 52 (August 1, 1978): 18.

LABOR ORGANIZATION

General

Amos, James L. Comparison of Measures Deployed by Unions to
Organize Ohio's Hospitals. Washington, D.C.: George Washington University, School of Government and Business Administration, 1970.

Amundson, Norman E. "Labor Relations and the Nursing Leader:
Union Dogma." Journal of Nursing Administration 4 (January-
February 1974): 14-15.

Berkeley, A. Eliot, ed. Labor Relations in Hospitals and Health
Care Facilities: Proceedings of a Conference Presented by the
American Arbitration Association and the Federal Conciliation
Service. Washington, D.C.: Bureau of National Affairs, 1976.

Bernard, J. "Organizing Hospital Workers." Working Papers 4
(Fall 1976): 53-59.

Bloem, Ruth S. "Collective Bargaining: What's It All About and What Can It Do for You?" Journal of Practical Nursing 25 (March 1975): 30-31, (April 1975): 26-27, and (May 1975): 22-23.

Bye, Basil, and Keith Jerrome. "Training the Hospital Union Steward." Hospital and Health Services Review 68 (April 1972): 116-17.

Davis, Leon J. "Local 1199 Union Power Plus Soul Power." New Physician 20 (May 1971): 313-17.

Davis, Leon J., and Elliott Godoff. "A National Hospital Union?" Hospital World 1 (October 1972): 13-17.

DeFriase, Gordon H. "Hospital Social Structure, the Professional Nurse, and Patient Care: A Study of Alienation from the Work Role." Ph.D. dissertation, University of Kentucky, 1967.

Dicker, Kathleen. "Unions vs. Colleges." Nursing Mirror 139 (October 24, 1974): 39.

Engle, G. V., and M. L. Schulman. "The Relationship of Unionization to Professionalism in Medicine." Journal of Medical Education 51 (February 1976): 132-34.

"50,000 Leaflets Assail Unions' Mail Prescription Plan." American Druggist 160 (July 28, 1969): 23.

"Florida 'Guild' Will Resemble Union." American Medical News 15 (May 22, 1972): 1.

Francke, Don E. "Economic Benefits and a Professional Society." Drug Intelligence and Clinical Pharmacy 4 (March 1970): 59.

Freeman, J. R. "You Can Too Learn to Live with Unions." Modern Hospital 103 (November 1964): 95-98.

Goldberg, Joel H. "Will House Staff Associations Become More Than Unions?" Hospital Physician 7 (June 1971): 59-60.

Gordon, Max. "Emancipating the Mental Wards." The Nation, December 16, 1968, pp. 650-53.

Grandre, L. de. "American Medical Unionism: Does Patient or Third Party Retain the Doctor?" Canadian Medical Association Journal 109 (October 20, 1973): 800.

"Health Care Unions Fare Better than Average." Hospital Personnel Administration 13 (June 1977): 1.

"Hospital Union Officials Indicted." Hospital Personnel Administration 9 (October 1973): 2.

"Hospital Union Wins Medical Center Vote." AFL-CIO News 22 (July 16, 1977): 7.

"In Union There Is What?" Kansas Medical Society Journal 73 (August 1972): 379-80.

Kirkland, L. "Labor's Point of View on HMOs." Public Health Report 90 (March-April 1975): 104-5.

Krekel, S. "The Union's Role in Occupational Health." Occupational Health Nurse (New York) 24 (October 1976): 13-14.

Lemmer, William P. "A Professional Society or a Trade Union as a Collective Bargaining Agent: 'What's the Difference?'" Michigan Hospitals 6 (June 1970): 2.

Levin, Tom. "Unions, Community and Enlightened Professionals: A New Alliance for Health Career Education." New Physician 20 (May 1971): 300-11.

Marcus, S. A. "The Purposes of Unionization in the Medical Profession: The Unionized Profession's Perspective in the United States." International Journal of Health Services 5 (1975): 37-42.

"Mental Health Employees' Rights as Seen by the American Federation of State, County and Municipal Employees." In Paper Victories and Hard Realities, edited by Valerie Bradley and Gary Clarke, pp. 134-40. Washington, D.C.: Health Policy Center, 1976. WM30, P214, 1975.

Metzger, Norman. "The Six Forms of Union Security." Hospital Management 112 (September 1971): 11.

Milliken, Ralph A., and Gerry Milliken. "Vulnerable and Outbid." Hospitals 47 (October 16, 1973): 56-59.

Mitchell, Keith. "The Role of Labor." National Hospital 14 (September 1970): 29-34.

Morgan, Jerry L. "Is Unionization Inevitable?" Newsletter of Hospital Personnel Administrators 8 (November 1972): 2-3.

"Not to Harm the Patient." Hospital and Health Services Review 70 (February 1974): 40-41.

Oswald, Rudy. "Voice for Hospital Workers." American Federationist 82 (January 1975): 14-17.

Sloan, Stanley. "Democracy in a Public Employee Union." Public Personnel Review 30 (October 1969): 194-98.

Stanton, Erwin S. "Unions and the Professional Employee." Hospital Progress 55 (January 1974): 58.

"State-County Adds 8,400 in Missouri." AFL-CIO News 22 (October 8, 1977): 2.

"Union Challenges ANA Education Programs." Association of Operating Room Nurses Journal 19 (February 1974): 560.

"Unthinkable No Longer: The Unionizing Ideal." Medical Economics 49 (April 10, 1972): 10-11.

Van Dellen, T. R. "Are Medical Unions Inevitable?" Illinois Medical Journal 142 (October 1972): 433.

Trends and Status

Abelow, William J. "Labor Forecast: More Unions, More Government Control." Modern Hospital 119 (November 1972): 64-65.

"Again It's NAGE Clobbering AFGE." Federal News 14 (March 1977): 1.

Alutto, Joseph A., and James A. Belasco. "Determinants of Attitudinal Militancy among Nurses and Teachers." Industrial and Labor Relations Review 27 (January 1974): 216.

Bairstow, F. "Professionalism and Unionism: Are They Compatible?" Industrial Engineering 6 (April 1974): 40-42.

Bellaby, P., et al. "The Growth of Trade Union Consciousness among General Hospital Nurses Viewed as a Response to 'Proletarianisation'." Sociological Review 25 (November 1977): 801-22.

Bullough, Bonnie. "The New Militancy in Nursing." Nursing Forum 10 (1971): 273-77.

"Can a Professional Association Be a Trade Union, Too?" Hospitals 48 (September 1, 1974): 103.

Chamot, D. "Professional Employees Turn to Unions." Harvard Business Review 54 (May-June 1976): 119-27.

Clark, G. M. "The Unionization of Hospital Professionals." Personnel 47 (July 1970): 40-46.

Coleman, Vernon. "Can Anyone Be a Health Professional and a Trade Unionist?" Nursing Mirror 139 (August 30, 1974): 41.

Davis, Leon J., and Moe Foner. "Organization and Unionization of Health Workers in the United States: The Trade Union Perspective." International Journal of Health Service 5 (1975): 19-26.

"Delegates See No Need for Union-Type Actions." American Medical News 15 (July 3, 1972): 8.

Denton, J. A. "Attitudes toward Alternative Models of Unions and Professional Associations." Nurse Resident 25 (May-June 1976): 178-80.

"Despite Hospital Hierarchy: Health Workers Unionize." Dollars & Sense: A Monthly Bulletin of Economic Affairs 15 (March 1976): 12-13.

"Doctors, Diplomats, Engineers: Trend to Professional Unions." U.S. News and World Report, June 5, 1972, pp. 100-2.

"Doctors, Nurses, Teachers—Why More Are Joining Unions." U.S. News and World Report, November 10, 1975, pp. 61-62.

Donovan, L. "Is Nursing Ripe for a Union Explosion?" RN 41 (May 1978): 62-65.

Engle, G. V., and M. L. Schulman. "The Relationship of Unionization to Professionalism in Medicine." Journal of Medical Education 51 (February 1976): 132-34.

Feitelberg, Samuel B. "A Professional Association Faces up to the Union Problem." American Journal of Hospital Pharmacy 27 (March 1970): 203-8.

Frederick, Larry D. "New Image for the AMA." Modern Health Care (February 1976): 160-61.

Gershenfeld, Walter. "Hospitals." In Emerging Sectors of Collective Bargaining, edited by Seymour Wolfbein, pp. 173-218. Morristown, N.J.: General Learning Press, 1970.

Grand, Norma K. "Nightingaleism, Employeeism, and Professional Collectivism." Nursing Forum 10 (1971): 289-99.

_____. "Nursing Ideologies and Collective Bargaining." Journal of Nursing Administration 3 (March-April 1973): 29-32.

"Hospitals Workers—A Militant New Force in Organized Labor." U.S. News and World Report, December 30, 1974, pp. 61-62.

"House Staff to Organize Nationally." American Medical News 14 (March 29, 1971): 1.

"Industrial Union Precedents Spread to Health Care Industry." Hospital Practice 10 (August 1975): 111-14.

Lombardi, V., and A. J. Grimes. "A Primer for a Theory of White Collar Unionization." Monthly Labor Review 90 (May 1967): 46-49.

Marcus, S. A. "The Purposes of Unionization in the Medical Profession: The Unionized Profession's Perspective in the United States." International Journal of Health Services 5 (1975): 37-42.

Matlack, David R. "Goals and Trends in the Unionization of Health Professionals." Hospital Progress 53 (February 1972): 32-33.

Miller, Jon D., and Stephen Shortell III. "Hospital Unionization: A Study of the Trends." Hospitals 43 (August 16, 1969): 67-73.

Munger, Mary D. "ANA Program to Promote Collective Bargaining." Hospital Topics 52 (May 1974): 23-24.

Myers, Morris L. "Professional Trade Unions." Hospitals 44 (August 16, 1970): 80-83.

Oswald, Rudy. "Voice for Hospital Workers." American Federationist 82 (January 1975): 14-17.

Petersen, D. J. "Labor Trends: White Collar Unionization and the Pay Board." Personnel 49 (July-August 1972): 34-39.

Pointer, Dennis D., and Lloyd Cannedy. "Organizing of Professionals: Associations Serve Union Function." Hospitals 46 (March 16, 1972): 70-73.

"Prescription Plan Pits Union against Union." American Druggist 159 (May 5, 1969): 28.

Rehmus, Charles M. "Unionism Inevitable for Some . . . An Alternative for Others." Michigan Hospitals 6 (March 1970): 23-24.

Richmond, Charles A. The Nature of Hospital Unions: An Evaluation of the Movement and Management's Reaction to It. Philadelphia: Temple University, 1971.

Selden, William K. "Professional Associations—Their Primary Functions." Journal of Allied Health 1 (November 1972): 25-28.

Stanton, Erwin S. "Unions and the Professional Employee." Hospital Progress 55 (January 1974): 58.

"Study Finds Union Activity on Increase in Hospitals." Hospitals 45 (August 16, 1971): 110-11.

Ten Boer, Martin H. "Study of the Extent and Impact of Organized Labor in Colleges and Universities." Ed.D. dissertation, Indiana University, 1970. Also in Journal of the College and University Personnel Association 22 (December 1970): 27-73.

"Trade Union Membership." Hospital Management 33 (January-February 1970): 13.

"Unions for Doctors Are Growing Trend." Management Digest 9 (June 22, 1972): 2-4.

Wurf, Jerry. "Revolution in the Public Sector." Hospital and Community Psychiatry 22 (April 1974): 17-19.

Professional Employees

Physicians

"AFL-CIO Affiliation 'Essential,' MD Unions Say." American Medical News 16 (January 15, 1973): 14.

Alper, Philip R. Doctors' Unions and Collective Bargaining. Report of Proceedings Conference of the Institute of Industrial Relations and American Federation of Physicians and Dentists, 1974, at the University of California at Berkeley.

"AMA Chief Says MD Unionism Violates Medical Ethics." Skin and Allergy News, August 1972, p. 40.

Andrews, Mary A. "Housestaff Physicians and Interns Press for Bargaining Rights." Monthly Labor Review 101 (August 1978): 30.

"As MD Unions Grow, So Does AMA's Dismay." Medical World News 13 (July 14, 1972): 18-19.

Balliett, Gene. "Doctors' Unions: The Economics of Muscle." Physician's Management 13 (August 1973): 27.

Barton, Walter E. "Physicians' Unions." Psychiatric News 9 (September 5, 1973): 2.

Bognanno, Mario F., James B. Dworkin, and Omatayo Fashoyin. "Physicians' and Dentists' Bargaining Organizations: A Preliminary Look." Monthly Labor Review 98 (June 1975): 33-35.

Bottone, Anthony. "Doctors' Unions: They're Here Right Now." Medical Opinion, July 1972, pp. 14-19.

Burton, Kenneth F. "The Case for a Doctors' Union Now." Medical Economics 49 (January 3, 1972): 103.

Chamot, D. "Professional Employees Turn to Unions." Harvard Business Review 54 (May-June 1976): 119-27.

"Delegates Oppose Physician's Unions." American Medical News 16 (July 2/9, 1973): 1.

"Doctors Forming Unions!" Perspective 7 (Third Quarter): 16-18.

"Doctors New Bag Out West Is Unionism." Medical World News 13 (April 14, 1972): 17-18.

"Doctors of the World . . . Unite?" Physician's Management 12 (August 1973): 27-34.

"Doctors, Trustees, and Unions." Modern Health Care, Short-Term Care Edition 2 (October 1974): 87.

"Doctors' Unions: The Economics of Muscle." Physician's Management 13 (August 1973): 27-34.

"Doctors, Unite!" Time, December 3, 1973, p. 86.

Downey, Gregg W. "Occupational Health Issue May Be Rallying Point for Doctors and Unions." Modern Hospital 118 (February 1972): 39-41.

Everist, Bruce W. "Physicians and Unions." Hospital Medical Staff 1 (August 1972): 1-2.

Ferber, Stanley. "Doctors' Unions—Down and Out?" Medical Economics 50 (September 17, 1973): 45.

Frederick, Larry D. "New Image for the AMA." Modern Health Care 5 (February 1976): 16K-L.

Kircher, William L. "Big Labor Cautions Doctors on Collective Bargaining." Medical Economics 49 (August 14, 1972): 80-87.

"Las Vegas MDs Form AFL-CIO Union." American Medical News 15 (April 3, 1972): 1.

"MDs Set up Three More AFL-CIO Locals." American Medical News 16 (January 8, 1973): 1.

Middleton, John. "Will Doctors Go the Union Route?" Medical Economics 48 (October 11, 1971): 154-55.

"More and More New York Doctors Join Professional Unions." New York Medicine 30 (1974): 54.

"National MD Union Awaits Locals' OK." American Medical News 15 (December 11, 1972): 1.

"National MD Union Planned." American Medical News 15 (November 6, 1972): 10.

"New Jersey MDs Reject Union, Set up Foundation." American Medical News 15 (May 22, 1972): 1-9.

Noie, Mancie. "Doctors Move beyond Medicine." Hospitals 50 (April 1, 1976): 69-72.

"Physicians Unions—Guilds ?" California Medicine 117 (September 1972): 92–95.

"Physicians Unions: House Staffs Organize." Medical World News 15 (December 20, 1974): 8.

Pointer, Dennis D., and Lloyd L. Cannedy. "Organizing of Professionals: Associations Serve Union Function." Hospitals 46 (March 16, 1972): 70–73.

"Salaried MDs Vote for Unionism." American Medical News 17 (November 8, 1974): 17.

"San Francisco Doctors Form Union and Identify Friends and Enemies." Modern Hospital 118 (June 1972): 46.

Schwartz, Harry. "The Changing Compact between American Doctors and Society." Modern Medicine 43 (June 15, 1975): 32–41.

"Six Groups Join National Physicians' Union." American Medical News 16 (February 5, 1973): 3.

"Special Report on Physician's Unions: What Are They . . . Recent Developments . . . Legal Aspects." Delaware Medical Journal 45 (February 1973): 44–48.

Steele, Mark M. "AMA Teaches Physicians to Fight Back." Modern Health Care 6 (July 1976): 31.

"The Unionizing Push in the Professions." Nation's Business 60 (November 1972): 39–42.

"Thirty Nevada Physicians Organize AFL-CIO Union." Internal Medicine News, May 1, 1972, p. 1.

Ulrich, Sylvia. "Physicians' Unions." Federation of American Hospitals Review 6 (April 1973): 32–37.

_____. "Will Your Appendectomy Be Performed by a Member of the AFL-CIO?" Modern Hospital 121 (October 1973): 63–65.

"Union Claims 1,000 MDs." American Medical News 17 (January 14, 1974): 9.

"Unionism Attractive to Many Physicians." Oklahoma State Medical Association Journal 65 (August 1972): 355.

"Unions for Physicians?" Journal of Dental Education 36 (October 1972): 11.

Registered Nurses

"ANA's Economic and General Welfare Program: Organizing the Local Unit." American Nursing Association Publication EC-133 (1975): 1-12.

"American Nurses' Association Contests Union Bid to Represent VA Nurses at National Level." American Journal of Nursing 71 (October 1971): 1874-75.

Anderson, Norman E. "Labor Relations and the Nursing Leader (Will the Supervisor Issue Destroy the Nurses' Association as a Professional Organization?)" Journal of Nursing Administration 3 (July-August 1973): 6.

Baird, William M. "Collective Bargaining by Registered Nurses." Ph.D. dissertation, Ohio State University, 1968.

Bullough, Bonnie. "The New Militancy in Nursing." Nursing Forum 10 (1971): 273-88.

DiMercurio, Gary M. Role Expectations of Registered Nurses as a Consequence of Unionization. Berkeley: Graduate Program in Hospital Administration, University of California, 1967.

Duran, T. "Professional Status and Economic Security." Vermont Registered Nurse 3 (June 1971): 6.

Epstein, Richard, et al. "The Nurse as a Professional and as a Unionist." Hospitals 50 (January 16, 1976): 44-48.

Evagorov, Deanna. "All for One and One for All." Nursing Times 67 (July 22, 1971): 904-5.

Godfrey, M. "Someone Should Represent Nurses." Nursing '76 6 (June 1976): 73.

Grand, K. N. "The Role of Ideology in the Unionization of Nurses."
Abstracts of Hospital Management Studies 9. Cleveland: Case
Western Reserve University, 1973.

Grand, Norma K. "Nursing Ideologies and Collective Bargaining."
Journal of Nursing Administration 3 (March–April 1973): 29–32.

Handel, David. Nurses and Collective Bargaining. Chicago: University of Chicago Press, 1969.

Hanson, Susan G. "Should Nurses Use Collective Bargaining?"
Association of Operating Room Nurses Journal 19 (January 1974):
23–24.

Hawley, Karen S. Economics of Collective Bargaining by Nurses.
Ames: Industrial Relations Center, Iowa State University,
September 1967.

Jacox, Ada. The Nurse's Cap: A Case Study of Administrator
Nurse Conflict. Cleveland: Case Western Reserve University,
1969.

Judge, Diane. "The New Nurse: A Sense of Duty and Testing."
Modern Health Care, Short-Term Care Edition 2 (October 1974):
21–27.

Klassen, Kathryn L. "Nurse's Right for Self-Determination in Professional Practice: Report from Kansas." Nursing Forum 10
(1971): 322–31.

Kruger, D. H. "Bargaining and the Nursing Profession." Monthly
Labor Review 84 (July 1961): 699–705.

Larkins, Eddie L. "Study of Grievances, 1971–1973, University
Hospital, Ann Arbor, Michigan." Master's thesis, University
of Michigan, 1974.

Mauksch, I. G. "Attainment of Control over Professional Practice."
Nursing Forum 10 (1971): 232–38.

McEvey, P. "Unionization or Professionalization: Which Way for
Nurses?" Nursing Mirror 141 (November 20, 1975): 70–72.

Meyer, G. Dale. "Determinants of Collective Action Attitudes
among Hospital Nurses: An Empirical Test of a Behavioral
Model." Ph.D. dissertation, University of Iowa, 1970.

Mignerey, D. "A New Challenge for RNs." Colorado Nurse 76 (November 1976): 4.

Munger, Mary D. "ANA Program to Promote Collective Bargaining." Hospital Topics 52 (May 1974): 23-24.

Nursing in Minnesota. Minneapolis: University of Minnesota, 1973.

Phillips, Donald F. "New Demands on Nurses." Hospitals 48 (September 16, 1974): 41-44.

Raney, James E. "Social Identity Factors as a Function of Nursing Attitudes toward Labor Organizations." Ph.D. dissertation, Washington University, 1970.

Reinhart, Robert S. "Communicating: Coping with Change." Association of Operating Room Nurses Journal 14 (January 1972): 41-48.

Schraeder, Elinor S. "Who Should Represent Nurses at the Bargaining Table?" Association of Operating Room Nurses Journal 19 (April 1974): 785-86.

Seidman, Joel. "Nurses and Collective Bargaining." Industrial and Labor Relations Review 23 (April 1970): 335-51.

Swanberg, Gloria. "Nursing/Labor Negotiating." Hospitals 44 (August 1, 1970): 54-56.

"The ANA: Can a Professional Association be a Trade Union, Too?" Hospitals 48 (September 1, 1974): 103.

Other Professionals

"ASHP Postpones Decision on Unionization." Hospitals 44 (June 16, 1970): 73-74.

Baumgartner, R. P. "Hospital Pharmacy Is Seen Facing Wave of Unionism." American Druggist 170 (September 1, 1974): 64-66.

Bowles, Grover. "Hospital Pharmacists Take First Step toward Active Collective Bargaining." Modern Hospital 116 (May 1971): 118-19.

Choich, Rudolph, Jr., and C. D. Hepler. "Factors Related to Collective Bargaining Preferences among Hospital Pharmacists." American Journal of Hospital Pharmacy 31 (May 1974): 456-66.

Cooper, Ben F. "Editorial on Pharmacist Unions." Hospital Pharmacy 5 (February 1970): 5-6.

Francke, Don E. "Meeting the Challenge of Change." American Journal of Hospital Pharmacy 27 (March 1970): 188-99.

Gruberg, L. "Are Guilds the Answer to Economic Security for Pharmacists?" American Druggist 160 (August 11, 1969): 16.

"Guild Represents 30 Mail Order Pharmacists." American Druggist 164 (December 13, 1971): 20.

Hidde, A. John, and Tim R. Lovington. "ASHP Members View Collective Bargaining." American Journal of Hospital Pharmacy 30 (May 1973): 428-35.

"Hospital Pharmacists Must Form Their Own Unions." American Druggist 160 (October 20, 1969): 32-33.

"How Unionism in Pharmacy Will Affect You." American Druggist Merchandising 168 (October 1, 1973): 22-24.

Kushner, D. "Piece of the Action." American Druggist 160 (December 15, 1969): 8-12.

"Pace of Union Drives Intensifies." American Druggist 161 (February 9, 1970): 20.

Rayburn, John M. "Professionalism and Pharmacy Unionism." Journal of the American Pharmaceutical Association NS11 (October 1971): 541-44.

"Report of Unionization of Hospital Pharmacists and the American Society of Hospital Pharmacists." American Journal of Hospital Pharmacy 26 (September 1969): 500-18.

"Retail Clerks Union Seeks to Organize All Arizona Pharmacists." American Druggist 160 (December 15, 1969): 16.

Roberts, Carl. "Pharmacy Unions—Misconceptions." Journal of the American Pharmaceutical Association NS10 (February 1970): 93-95.

Schowalter, Joyce M., and Lynda F. Cole. Nurse Power in Minnesota. St. Paul: Northlands Regional Medical Programs, 1971.

Shaw, Clayton R. "Professionalism—A Sociological Evaluation of Commercialism and Inconsistencies in Pharmacy." Journal of the American Pharmaceutical Association NS11 (October 1971): 539.

Teplitsky, Benjamin. "What Chief Hospital Rx Men Think about Unions." Pharmacy Times 37 (February 1971): 46–53.

"Union Role Is Urged for ASHP." American Druggist 161 (January 1970): 26–28.

Technical Employees

Barnes, David L. "Collective Bargaining for Radiologic Technologists: Organizational Vehicles." Radiologic Technology 46 (January–February 1975): 282–93.

Brodeur, Armand E. "Future Technologists: Unionism, Professionalism, or Licensure?" Radiologic Technology 5 (March 1970): 280–83.

Doppelt, Lawrence. "Unions and Your Hospital: A Practical Guide for Radiologists." Practical Radiology 1 (February 1973): 23–24.

Dyson, R. "Should Physiotherapists Join Trade Unions?" Physiotherapy 61 (October 1975): 302–4.

Farley, Marilyn. "When Technologists Join Unions." Applied Radiology, June/July 1972, p. 23.

Liverett, James A. "Unions, Licensure, Education, and Reorganization." Respiratory Care 16 (September–October 1971): 205–11.

Sandoz, Ruth L. "Technologists, Unions and the N.E.C." Radiologic Technology 46 (November–December 1974): 200–2.

Nonprofessional Employees

McKersie, Robert B., and Montague Brown. "Nonprofessional Hospital Workers and a Union Organizing Drive." Quarterly Journal of Economics, August 1963, pp. 372–404.

"Paraprofessionals React to Labor Union Efforts and May Set up a Nationwide Bargaining Unit." Modern Hospital 119 (September 1972): 41–42.

LABOR-MANAGEMENT RELATIONS AND CONFLICT

General

"A Hospital's Policy on Unions." Personnel Policy Briefs, September 1, 1973, p. 1.

"A.S.H.P. Counsel Sees Benefits in Union Role." American Druggist 100 (December 15, 1964): 20.

Alutto, Joseph A., and James A. Belasco. "Determinants of Attitudinal Militancy among Nurses and Teachers." Industrial and Labor Relations Review 27 (January 1974): 216–27.

"American Society for Medical Technology Position Statement on Collective Bargaining and Position Definitions." American Journal of Medical Technologists 42 (May 8, 1976): 42.

Amos, James L. Comparison of Measures Deployed by Unions to Organize Ohio's Hospitals. Washington, D.C.: George Washington University, School of Government and Business Administration, March 1970.

Amundson, Norman E. "Labor Relations and the Nursing Leader." Journal of Nursing Administration 2 (May–June 1972): 10.

Analysis of Collective Bargaining Agreements in Chicago Area Hospitals 1975-1976. Chicago: Chicago Hospital Council, Employee/Labor Relations Services, 1976.

"Associations Mount Anti-Union Drive." American Druggist 161 (February 23, 1970): 15.

Bailey, Jack C. A Comparative Study of the Employment Conditions of Nurses (With and without Collective Bargaining). Washington, D.C.: George Washington University, June 1965.

Balliett, Gene. "Doctors' Unions: The Economics of Muscle." Physician's Management 13 (August 1973): 27.

Baltch, Philip R. Unions in Hospitals. Cincinnati: Xavier University, 1968.

Becker, Brian E. "The Impact of Unions on Labor Costs in Hospitals: A Three State Study." Ph.D. dissertation, University of Wisconsin at Madison, 1977.

Bennett, Addison C. "Resisting Union Organizing Attempts." Hospital Topics 50 (January 1972): 30-34.

Best, Robert. "How the Technologist Views 'Management'." Practical Radiology 1 (February 1973): 10-18.

"Bid Win at Cook County Hospital." Service Employee 22 (October 1971): 2.

Bloem, Ruth S. "Collective Bargaining: What's It All about and What Can It Do for You?" Journal of Practical Nursing 25 (March 1975): 30-31, (April 1975): 26-27, and (May 1975): 22-23.

Bloom, B. I. "Collective Action by Professionals Poses Problems for Administrators." Hospitals 51 (March 16, 1977): 167.

Boss, Donna. "Management vs. Labor, 'We Want More Work!'" Food Management 10 (February 1975): 36.

Boyer, John M., Carl Westerhaus, and John Coggeshall. Employee Relations and Collective Bargaining in Health Care Facilities. 2d ed. St. Louis: C. V. Mosby, 1975.

Brand, I. A. G. "Function of Employer Organizations." National Hospital 16 (September 1972): 25-32.

Brigden, Raymond J. "Industrial Relations." Supervisor Nurse 3 (February 1972): 19-21.

Brothers, P. E. Collective Bargaining by Nurses under the American Nurses' Association's Economic Security Program: An Historical and Empirical Description. Iowa City: University of Iowa, 1972.

Bunker, Charles S. Collective Bargaining: Non-Profit Sector. Columbus: Grid, 1973.

Cargo, J. W. "Advantages/Disadvantages of Labor Unions in the Health Care Institutions." Hospital Management 111 (June 1971): 22.

Carlson, D. R. "Labor Union: Color It White, Black, or Red." Modern Hospital 105 (August 1965): 107-11.

Cassell, Frank H. "The Direction of Labor-Management in the United States Health Sector." British Journal of Industrial Relations 14 (March 1976): 18-25.

Centner, J. L. "Hospitals and Collective Bargaining." Personnel Journal 38 (November 1959): 203-5.

Christopher, W. I. "Hospitals and Unions Come to Grips." Hospital Topics 52 (May 1974): 21-24.

"Chronology of a Hospital Union Campaign." Hospital Topics 54 (March-April 1976): 53-58.

Clark, G. M. "The Unionization of Hospital Professionals." Personnel 47 (July 1970): 40-46.

Cleland, Virginia S. "To End Sex Discrimination." Nursing Clinics of North America 9 (September 1974): 563-71.

"Collective Agreements in Hospitals." Labor Gazette 66 (July 1966): 354-55.

Conta, Lionne. "Bargaining by Professionals." American Journal of Nursing 72 (February 1972): 309-12.

Crouch, Winston W. "Local Government Labor Relations Today." Public Management 57 (February 1975): 4-6.

"Current Trends in Industrial Relations—Areas of Concern." Midwives Chronicle 91 (July 1978): 170.

Dabney, Henrietta L. "Discussion of Attitudes on Hospitals and Collective Bargaining." In Proceedings of the Twenty-Second Annual Winter Meeting of the Industrial Relations Research Association, edited by Gerald G. Somers, pp. 226-34. Madison: Industrial Relations Research Association, 1969.

Davis, Leon J. "Local 1199 Union Power Plus Soul Power." New Physician 20 (May 1971): 313-17.

"Despite Hospital Hierarchy: Health Workers Unionize." Dollars and Sense: A Monthly Bulletin of Economic Affairs 15 (March 1976): 12-13.

Dickenson, M. "Administrative Problems in Union Organizations."
Royal Australian Nursing Federation Review 6 (May 1975): 7.

Dicker, Kathleen. "Unions vs. Colleges." Nursing Mirror 139
(October 24, 1974): 39.

DiMercurio, Gary M. Role Expectations of Registered Nurses as a
Consequence of Unionization. Berkeley: University of California,
Graduate Program in Hospital Administration, 1967.

Edwards, Kimberly, and Susan P. Mahan. "Organized Labor in
Non-Profit Agencies." The American Journal of Occupational
Therapy 24 (March 1970): 128-31.

"Effects of Unionization Stir Concern." American Medical News 17
(August 26, 1974): 1.

Ehrenreich, B., and J. H. Ehrenreich. "Hospital Workers: Class
Conflicts in the Making." International Journal of Health Services 5 (1975): 43-51.

Employee/Labor Relations Activity in Michigan Hospitals, December
31, 1973. Michigan Hospital Association, Report no. 40, n.d.
(1974).

Employee/Labor Relations Activity in Michigan Hospitals, June 30,
1974. Michigan Hospital Association, Report no. 42, n.d. (1974).

Employment and Conditions of Work and Life of Nursing Personnel.
Report 7, Part 2, Sixty-First Session of the International Labour
Conference, Geneva, 1976.

Erb, Alma. "Labor Unions and Their Effect on Health Care Institutions." Executive Housekeeper 20 (June 1973): 62.

Erickson, Eva H. "Collective Bargaining: An Inappropriate Technique for Professionals." Nursing Forum 10 (1971): 300-1.

"Factors That Make Employees Union-Prone." Hospital Engineering
19 (November-December 1974): 5-6.

Faine, Jeffry C. The Extent and Impact of Collective Bargaining
and Unionization upon the Nonprofit Hospital. Washington, D.C.:
George Washington University, Department of Health Care Administration, School of Government and Business Administration,
December 1970.

"Financial Incentives Invalidate Union Election." Newsletter of the American Society of Hospital Attorneys 6 (March 1973): 3-4.

Foster, J. T. "Roving Report. Good Story Well Told Defeats Two Union Efforts at Wisconsin Hospital." Modern Hospital 103 (July 1964): 36-39.

Fox, Thomas G. "Medical School Faculty Factors Influencing Disposition to Collective Bargaining." Journal of Medical Education 50 (March 1975): 229-36.

Francke, Don E. "Economic Benefits and a Professional Society." Drug Intelligence and Clinical Pharmacy 4 (March 1970): 59.

_____. "Meeting the Challenge of Change." American Journal of Hospital Pharmacy 27 (March 1970): 188-99.

Frenzen, P. D. "Survey Updates Unionization Activities." Hospitals 52 (August 1, 1978): 93.

Gershenfeld, Walter. "Hospitals." In Emerging Sectors of Collective Bargaining, edited by Seymour Wolfbein, pp. 173-218. Morristown, N.J.: General Learning Press, 1970.

Giovannetti, R. J. "What Groups of Employees Will the Union Attempt to Organize?" Journal of the American Health Care Association 3 (July 1977): 5.

Goldstein, Stephen B. The Effect of an Imposed Union Organization on Attitudes toward Union by Psychologists in the New York State Department of Mental Hygiene. St. Louis: Washington University, 1972.

Goodfellow, Matthew. "Checklist on Susceptibility to Union: How Organizer Rates Your Hospital." Hospital Topics 51 (January 1973): 33-36.

_____. "How the Union Organizer Rates Your Facility." Nursing Homes, December-January 1974, pp. 7-11.

Gordon, Max. "Emancipating the Mental Wards." The Nation, December 16, 1968, pp. 650-53.

Grams, R. J. "Developing a Labor Relations Program." Hospital Forum 18 (May 1976): 6.

214 / COLLECTIVE BARGAINING AND HOSPITALS

Grant, R. A. "Unions Exist Because of Management's Short-Sightedness." Canadian Hospitals 50 (January 1973): 8.

Grossman, E. "Work Schedule and the Collective Agreement." Dimensions of Health Service 55 (July 1978): 38-39.

Hawley, Karen S. Economics of Collective Bargaining by Nurses. Ames: Iowa State University Press, 1967.

Hay, H. C. "Can You Keep a Union Out of Your Lab?" Medical Laboratory Observer 9 (October 1977): 43-46.

Heath, Richard M. "The Role of Union and Management in Public Psychiatric Hospitals." Journal of Health Administration 1 (Summer 1972): 15-22.

_____. "Union-Management Relations in Public Psychiatric Hospitals." Hospital and Community Psychiatry 21 (February 1970): 56-58.

Helin, E. B. "Chronology of a Hospital Union Campaign." Hospital Topics 54 (March-April 1976): 53-58.

Hepton, Estelle. Battle for the Hospitals: A Study of Unionization in Non-Profit Hospitals. Bulletin no. 49, Ithaca, N.Y.: New York State School of Industrial and Labor Relations, Cornell, 1963.

Herron, I., et al. "Labor-Management Issues in the Health Care Field." National League for Nursing Publications (1976): 1-59.

Hershey, Nathan. "Labor Relations in Hospitals in the Private Sector." In Proceedings of the Twenty-Second Annual Winter Meeting of the Industrial Relations Research Association, edited by Gerald G. Somers, pp. 217-25. Madison: Industrial Relations Research Association, 1969.

Herzog, Eric L. Work Relationship in the Delivery of Health Care: An Analysis of the Division of Labor between Physicians and Nurse Practitioners in Outpatient Clinics. Cambridge, Mass.: Massachusetts Institute of Technology, 1973. (Available from N.T.I.S.)

"Housestaff Organizing Activity, Development, Opponents." Hospital Physician 11 (October 1975): 8-15.

"How to Win the Labor Tug of War?" Modern Health Care, Short-Term Edition 2 (September 1974): 56-60.

Hunter, T. H. "Sounding Board: How Many Hats Can a House Officer Wear?" New England Journal of Medicine 294 (March 11, 1976): 608-9.

Jackson, L., et al. "Unions and the Facility: Why You Should Strive to Remain Free." American Health Care Association 2 (May 1976): 15-17.

Jacox, Ada. "Collective Bargaining in Academe." Nursing Outlook 21 (November 1973): 700-3.

_____. "Conflicting Loyalties in Collective Bargaining: An Empirical Illustration." Journal of Nursing Administration 1 (September-October 1971): 19-24.

"Join the Union and Win $50 an Hour for Review Work." Medical World News 13 (September 29, 1972): 17-18.

Juris, Hervey. "Labor Agreements in the Hospital Industry: A Study of Collective Bargaining Outputs." Labor Law Journal 28 (August 28, 1977): 504-11.

Kalman, Mervyn K. "Hospital Pharmacy and Economic Welfare: Where Do We Go from Here?" Hospital Pharmacy 5 (November 1970): 4-7.

Kassalow, E. M. "What Happens When Everyone Organizes?" Monthly Labor Review 95 (April 1972): 27-32.

Katz, Barbara F. "The Impact of Collective Bargaining on the Delivery of Health Care Services." Paper presented at the Annual Meeting of the American Public Health Association, November 17, 1975, in Chicago.

Keating, R. J. "Health Care Labor Relations Literature." Hospital Progress 58 (July 1977): 12-13.

Keaton, Harry J. "Labor Relations." Hospital Forum (Western) 13 (January 1971): 6.

Klassen, Kathryn L. "Nurse's Right for Self-Determination in Professional Practice: Report from Kansas." Nursing Forum 10 (1971): 322-31.

Kochery, David R., and George Strauss. "The Nonprofit Hospital and the Union." Buffalo Law Review, Winter 1960, pp. 255-82.

Kossoris, M. D. "San Francisco Bay Area Nurses' Negotiations." Monthly Labor Review 90 (June 1967): 8-12.

Kushner, D. "Piece of the Action." American Druggist 160 (December 15, 1969): 8-12.

"Labor Issues Affecting Health Care Institutions." Labor Relations Reporter, Background News and Information, May 26, 1975, pp. 89LRR80-89LRR83.

Labor-Management Issues in the Health Care Field. New York: National League for Nursing, 1976.

"Labor Relations Update." Hospitals 50 (October 1, 1976): 64.

Laner, Richard. "Employer-Employee Relations: Unions and Hospitals." Radiologic Technology 46 (July-August 1974): 10-19.

Ledbetter, B. E. "Labor Relations and the Nurse: An Overview." Oklahoma Nurse 20 (May 1975): 2.

"Let Employees Vote on Unionization, 1199 Official Tells Administrators." Modern Hospital 114 (May 1970): 42.

Lewis, H. L. "Separate Collective Bargaining." Modern Health Care 4 (July 1975): 51.

Lombardi, V., and A. J. Grimes. "A Primer for a Theory of White Collar Unionization." Monthly Labor Review 90 (May 1967): 46-49.

Mancano, John M. Nursing Staffs, Hospitals, and Industrial Relations. Washington, D.C.: George Washington University, 1967.

Marcus, Averill G. "Collective Bargaining in Nonprofit Hospitals." Industrial and Labor Relations Research 13 (May 1967): 3-12.

Match, Robert K., et al. "Unionization, Strikes, Threatened Strikes, and Hospitals—The View from Hospital Management." International Journal of Health Services 5 (1975): 27-36.

Matlack, David R. "Coping with the Unionization of Health Professionals." Hospital Progress 53 (March 1972): 32-36.

Mauksch, Ingeborg G. "Attainment of Control over Professional Practice." Nursing Forum 10 (1971): 232-38.

McCormick, William, Jr. "Labor Relations and Labor Costs in Hospitals." Ph.D. dissertation, Case Western Reserve University, 1968.

_____. "Labor Relations in Hospitals." American Journal of Nursing 70 (December 1970): 2606-9.

Menkes, J. J. Collective Bargaining in Voluntary Hospitals: Myth or Reality. Abstracts of Hospital Management Studies, vol. 10, no. 2. New York: City University of New York, 1974.

Metzger, Norman E. "Collective Bargaining and the Professional Employee." Hospital Administration 112 (April 1971): 10.

_____. "Coping with Unionization." Nursing Care 6 (October 1973): 24-27.

_____. "Despite Unionization, Administrators Can Control Policy, Cost, Quality." Hospital Progress 58 (September 1977): 36.

_____. "Labor Relations." Hospitals 44 (March 16, 1970): 80-84.

_____. "Preventive Labor Relations: Communication the Key." Hospital Progress 58 (April 1977): 79-82.

_____. "The Role of the Supervisor in the Unionization of Employees." Hospital Management 112 (August 1971): 10.

_____. "The Six Forms of Union Security." Hospital Management 112 (September 1971): 11.

Miller, R. U., et al. "Union Effects on Hospital Administration: Preliminary Results from a Three-State Study." Labor Law Journal 28 (August 1977): 512-19.

Miller, Ronald L. "Collective Bargaining: A New Frontier for Hospitals." Hospital Progress 56 (February 1975): 58.

_____. "The Hospital Union Relationship—Part 1." Hospitals 45 (May 1, 1971): 49-54.

_____. "The Hospital Union Relationship—Part 2." Hospitals 45 (May 16, 1971): 52-56.

Milliken, Ralph A., and Gerry Milliken. "Vulnerable and Outbid." Hospitals 47 (October 16, 1973): 56-59.

Mitchell, Keith. "The Role of Labor." National Hospital 14 (September 1970): 29-34.

Moore, T. F. "Union Decertification: Bucking the Trend." Hospital Topics 55 (May/June 1977): 14-15.

Munger, Mary D. "ANA Program to Promote Collective Bargaining." Hospital Topics 52 (May 1974): 23-24.

Nash, Al. "Hospital's Value System and the Union." Hospital Administration 19 (Fall 1974): 49-64.

_____. "Local 1199, Drug and Hospital Union: An Analysis of the Normative and Institutional Orders of a Complex Organization." Human Relations 27 (1974): 547-66.

"OR Nurse—Betwixt Union and Management." Hospitals 48 (May 1, 1974): 77-81.

Osterhaus, Leo B. "The Industrial Relations System in the Hospital Industry." Personnel Journal 47 (May 1968): 315-20, and (June 1968): 412-19.

Ottensmeyer, David J. "One Group Practice Faces up to Unions." Group Practice 23 (September–October 1974): 17.

"Pace of Union Drive Intensifies." American Druggist 161 (February 9, 1970): 20.

Phillips, Donald F. "Cook County Hospital: Politics and Power Plays." Hospitals 50 (March 16, 1976): 101-3.

Pointer, Dennis D. "Catholic Hospitals' Dual Nature Complicates Labor Relations Strategy." Hospital Progress 57 (February 1976): 58-61.

_____. "Employee Organization in Health Care Facilities: An Exploratory Analysis and Evaluation." Ph.D. dissertation, University of Iowa, 1971.

_____. Unionization, Collective Bargaining and the Nonprofit Hospital. College of Business Administration, Center for Labor and Management Monograph Series no. 13. Iowa City: University of Iowa, 1969.

Pointer, Dennis D., and Norman Metzger. Labor-Management Relations in the Health Services Industry: Theory and Practice. Washington, D.C.: Science and Health, 1972.

"Positions Funded for SNA Efforts." American Nurse 6 (April 1974): 1.

Powel, John Hare, Jr. "Theory of Union Behavior Applied to the Medical Profession." Ph.D. dissertation, University of Washington, 1973.

Provost, George P. "Collective Bargaining through Affiliated Chapters?" American Journal of Hospital Pharmacy 27 (March 1970): 187.

Rakich, Jonathan S. "Hospital Unionization: Causes and Effects." Hospital Administration 18 (Winter 1973): 7-18.

Rayburn, John M. "Barriers to Collective Bargaining in the Profession of Pharmacy." Hospital Pharmacy 5 (November 1970): 11-14.

Reece, D. A. "Union Decertification and the Salaried Approach: A Workable Alternative." Journal of Nursing Administration 7 (July-August 1977): 20-24.

"Revco Settles Strike but Bypasses Society." American Druggist 160 (December 15, 1969): 16.

Roth, Russell B. "Unions: Do They Unify or Divide?" American Medical News 16 (April 2, 1973): 4-5.

Sampson, Arthur J. "Labor Unions and the Nursing Home." Journal of the American College of Nursing Home Administrators 2 (Summer 1974): 37-46.

"San Francisco Doctors Form Union and Identify Friends and Enemies." Modern Hospital 118 (June 1972): 46.

"Season of Their Discontent: Unions Press Several Organizing Drives." Modern Hospital 114 (February 1970): 36C–36D.

Seidman, Joel. "Nurses and Collective Bargaining." Industrial and Labor Relations Review 23 (April 1970): 335–51.

Sellentin, Jerry L. "Labor's Concerns Face Management's." Hospitals 50 (April 1, 1976): 65–67.

Sibson, Robert E. "Why Unions in the Hospital?" Hospital Topics 43 (August 1965): 47–48.

Smith, David A. "Strike! Or—Why Not to Join a Union." Pennsylvania Medicine 76 (January 1973): 33.

Stempf, G. L. "Labor Relations among Professional Groups." Journal of the American Dietetic Association 65 (August 1974): 138–43.

Tambour, M. "Unions and Voluntary Agencies." Social Work 18 (July 1973): 41–47.

Terenzio, J. V. "What Every Administration Should Know—and Do—about Labor Relations." Hospitals 38 (August 1, 1964): 43–45.

"Try Group Practice to Stop Union." American Druggist 161 (March 9, 1970): 31.

"Union Gains Laid to Medical Society Failures." American Medical News 16 (February 26, 1973): 8.

"Union Organizers Appeal to the Discontent of Professionals." American Druggist 161 (January 26, 1970): 15.

"Union Teams up with Black Power." Business Week, April 5, 1969, pp. 22–24.

"Unionization and Right to Care May Be 'Gaining on' AHA." Hospital Practice, June 1972, p. 148.

"Unions in Hospitals." Southern Hospitals 41 (March 1973): 4.

"Unions Opposed." American Medical News 16 (April 30, 1973): 1–7.

Van Cleve, William J. "Collective Bargaining in the Health Care Industry." Journal of the American Dietetic Association 61 (December 1972): 633-36.

Vinci, Louis J. Unionization of Health Care Facilities in South Florida. Washington, D.C.: George Washington University, 1970.

Weimer, Edward W. "Hospitals and Unions Come to Grips." Hospital Topics 52 (May 1974): 21-23.

Weinmann, Richard A. "Unions: What Choice?" Cornell Hotel and Restaurant Administration 14 (August 1973): 13-15.

Werther, W. B. "Unions Do Not Happen, They Are Caused." National League for Nursing. Publication #20-1725. New York, 1978: 1-14.

Wood, C. K. "Industrial Relations in the Public Sector." National Hospital 18 (November 1974): 19-22.

"Your Opinion Please." Michigan Medicine 71 (November 1972): 956-58.

Negotiations: Structure, Practices, and Subjects

"ANA's Economic and General Welfare Program. Organizing the Local Unit." American Nursing Association Publication EC-133 (1975): 1-12.

Abelow, William J., and Norman Metzger. "Multi-Employer Bargaining for Health Care Institutions." Employee Relations Law Journal 1 (Winter 1976): 390-409.

Alper, Philip R., ed. Doctors' Unions and Collective Bargaining. Report of Proceedings Conference of the Institute of Industrial Relations and American Federation of Physicians and Dentists, 1974, at the University of California at Berkeley.

Anderson, Larry S. A Social Analysis of Bargaining between Hospitals and Registered Professional Nurses. Iowa City: Graduate Program in Hospital and Health Administration, University of Iowa, 1967.

Appelbaum, Alan L. "Third-Party Payers Gain Most from Arbitrated Labor Disputes." Hospitals, JAHA 50 (November 16, 1976): 72-76.

Baird, William M. "Collective Bargaining by Registered Nurses." Ph.D. dissertation, Ohio State University, 1968.

Barnes, David L. "Collective Bargaining for Radiologic Technologists: Organizational Vehicles." Radiologic Technology 46 (January-February 1975): 282-93.

"Bay Area Hospital Employees Win New Pacts." Service Employee 36 (June 1977): 3.

Bloem, Ruth S. "Collective Bargaining: What's It All About and What Can It Do for You?" Journal of Practical Nursing 25 (March 1975): 30-31, (April 1975): 26-27, and (May 1975): 22-23.

Bosanquet, Nicholas. "Words Can Win More Pay." Nursing Times 70 (February 21, 1974): 256-57.

Boyer, John M., Carl Westerhaus, and John Coggeshall. Employee Relations and Collective Bargaining in Health Care Facilities. 2d ed. St. Louis: C. V. Mosby, 1975.

Brothers, P. E. Collective Bargaining by Nurses under the American Nurses' Association's Economic Security Program: An Historical and Empirical Analysis. Iowa City: University of Iowa, 1972.

Bunker, Charles S. Collective Bargaining: Non-Profit Sector. Columbus: Grid, 1973.

Christopher, W. I. "Hospital and Unions Come to Grips." Hospital Topics 52 (May 1974): 21-24.

Cleland, Virginia S. "The Supervisor in Collective Bargaining." Journal of Nursing Administration 4 (1975): 33-35.

"Collective Bargaining." Hospital and Health Services Review 70 (April 1974): 141-43.

"Collective Bargaining and Unions for Doctors." Resident and Staff Physician 19 (July 1973): 54-59.

Conta, Lionne. "Bargaining by Professionals." American Journal of Nursing 72 (February 1972): 309-12.

Cook, Eugenia. "Collective Bargaining." Hospital Pharmacy Management 5 (March 1970): 16-18.

Dimmock, Stuart. "Collective Bargaining in the NHS." Health and Social Services Journal 84 (October 1974): 2292-93.

"Doctors' Unions: The Economics of Muscle." Physician's Management 13 (August 1973): 27-34.

Elkin, Randyl D. "Negotiating and Administrating a Union Contract." Hospital Progress 56 (January 1975): 40-43.

Faine, Jeffry C. The Extent and Impact of Collective Bargaining and Unionization upon the Non-Profit Hospital. Washington, D.C.: George Washington University, School of Government and Business Administration, December 1970.

Feuille, Peter, Charles Maxey, Hervey Juris, and Margaret Levi. "Determinants of Multi-Employer Bargaining in Hospitals." Employee Relations Law Journal 4 (Summer 1978): 98-115.

Fottler, Myron D. "The Union Impact on Hospital Wages." Industrial and Labor Relations Review 30 (April 1977): 342-55.

"Four-Day Workweek? Oh Those Long Weekends!" RN 35 (January 1972): 42-45.

Galvin, J. Michael, Jr. Collective Bargaining—Union Relations. Cincinnati: Xavier University, Graduate School of Hospital Administration, May 15, 1969.

Gamm, Sara. "Collective Bargaining in Non-Profit Hospitals." Industrial and Labor Relations Review 5 (1968): 12-13.

Gershenfeld, Walter. "Hospitals." In Emerging Sectors of Collective Bargaining, edited by Seymour Wolfbein, pp. 173-218. Morristown, N.J.: General Learning Press, 1970.

_____. "Organizing and Bargaining in Hospitals." Monthly Labor Review 91 (July 1968): 51-52.

Goodwin, Harold I., and Marie C. Vittetoe. "What Should Be the Role of Collective Bargaining for Medical Technologists?" Journal of Collective Negotiations 3 (Fall 1974): 317-25.

Gordon, Murray A. "Hospital Housestaff Collective Bargaining." Employee Relations Law Journal 1 (Winter 1976): 418-38.

Gruberg, L. "Ohio Pharmacists' Society Wants Higher Wages." American Druggist 159 (May 19, 1969): 19.

Hacker, John S. "Militant Actions by Nurses in Collective Bargaining in Voluntary Not-for-Profit Hospitals: An Exploratory Analysis." Master's thesis, University of Iowa, 1973.

Handel, David. Nurses and Collective Bargaining. Chicago: University of Chicago Press, 1969.

Hidde, A. John, and Tim R. Lovington. "ASHP Members View Collective Bargaining." American Journal of Hospital Pharmacy 30 (May 1973): 428-35.

Himmelsbach, William A. Toward a Game-Behavioral Mode for the Collective Bargaining Process and Its Implications in the Hospital Sector. Pittsburgh: University of Pennsylvania, Graduate School of Public Health, May 1970.

Hobart, C. L. "Collective Bargaining with Professionals: Conflict, Containment, or Accommodation?" Health Care Management Review 1 (Spring 1976): 7-16.

"Hospital Professionals Seek Joint Bargaining." Hospital World 1 (August 1972): 1.

"Hospitals Face Bargaining." America 118 (January 20, 1968): 66.

"Housestaff Organizing Activity, Development, Opponents." Hospital Physician 11 (October 1975): 8-15.

Howard, David L. "Views on A.S.H.P.'s Involvement in Collective Bargaining." American Journal of Hospital Pharmacy 27 (March 1970): 217-20.

Hush, Howard. "Collective Bargaining in Voluntary Agencies." Journal of Nursing Administration 1 (November-December 1971): 55-58.

"Industry's Nurses and Collective Bargaining." Occupational Health Nurse 19 (December 1971): 10-11.

Jacox, Ada. "Collective Action and Control of Practice by Professionals." Nursing Forum 10 (1971): 239-57.

_____. "Collective Bargaining in Academe." Nursing Outlook 21 (November 1973): 700-3.

_____. "Conflicting Loyalties in Collective Bargaining: An Empirical Illustration." Journal of Nursing Administration 1 (September-October 1971): 19-24.

Juris, Hervey. "Nationwide Survey Shows Growth in Union Contracts." Hospitals 51 (March 16, 1977): 122.

Kleingartner, Archie. "Collective Bargaining between Salaried Professional and Public Sector Management." Public Administration Review 33 (March-April 1973): 165-72.

Kossoris, M. D. "San Francisco Bay Area 1966 Nurses' Negotiations." Monthly Labor Review 90 (June 1967): 8-12.

Kralewski, J. E. "Collective Bargaining among Professional Employees." Hospital Administration 19 (1974): 30-41.

Kravit, Stan. "Collective Bargaining for Professionals." Supervisor Nurse 4 (July 1973): 46-51.

Kruger, D. H. "Bargaining and the Nursing Profession." Monthly Labor Review 84 (July 1961): 699-705.

Kushner, D. "Piece of the Action." American Druggist 160 (December 15, 1969): 8-12.

Lanzone, O. A. "The RN as Negotiator." Association of Operating Room Nurses Journal 22 (July 1975): 45-48.

Lewis, H. L. "Separate Collective Bargaining." Modern Health Care 4 (July 1975): 51.

"MD Union Signs First Contract [Las Vegas]." American Medical News 15 (October 2, 1972): 1.

Marcus, Averill G. "Collective Bargaining in Non-Profit Hospitals." Industrial and Labor Relations Research 13 (May 1967): 3-12.

Mauksch, Ingeborg G. "Attainment of Control over Professional Practice." Nursing Forum 10 (1971): 232-38.

Menkes, J. J. Collective Bargaining in the Voluntary Hospitals: Myth or Reality. Abstracts of Hospital Management Studies, vol. 10, no. 2. New York: City University of New York, 1974.

Metzger, Norman. "ANA Code Becoming Key Bargaining Issue for Nurses." Health/Labor Management Reports 3 (April 1973): 1.

_____. "Collective Bargaining and the Professional Employee." Hospital Administration 112 (April 1971): 10.

_____. "The Unique Nature of Voluntary Hospital Collective Bargaining." Executive Housekeeper 19 (May 1972): 38.

_____. "Whatever Happened to Collective Bargaining or the Dilemma of a Negotiator in the Hospital Industry." In Conference on Labor, New York University, Proceedings No. 27, pp. 87-92. New York: Bender, 1975.

_____. "You Must Learn to Do a New Dance Step . . . If You Are Negotiating a Contract with Nurses." Hospital Management 112 (May 1971): 10-11.

Miller, Ronald L. "Collective Bargaining in Nonprofit Hospitals." Ph.D. dissertation, University of Pennsylvania, 1969.

_____. "Development and Structure of Collective Bargaining among Registered Nurses." Personnel Journal 50 (February-March 1971): 134-40.

Milliken, Ralph A., and Gerry Milliken. "Vulnerable and Outbid." Hospitals 47 (October 16, 1973): 56-59.

Munger, Mary D. "ANA Program to Promote Collective Bargaining." Hospital Topics 52 (May 1974): 23-24.

"New Basis for Negotiations?" Health and Social Services Journal 83 (March 21, 1973): 720-21.

Norville, J., and R. J. Halonen. "Negotiating and Administering Contracts with Hospital-Based Physicians." Hospital Progress 56 (June 1975): 61-67.

"Occupational Health Nurses and Collective Bargaining." Occupational Health Nurse 25 (January 1977): 15-16.

"Ohio Association Sets up Negotiations Unit." American Druggist 159 (June 16, 1969): 19.

Packer, Clinton L. " 'Negotiations Book' Aids Management at Collective Bargaining Table." Hospital Topics 49 (August 1971): 40-43.

_____. Preparing Hospital Management for Labor Contract Negotiations. Chicago: American Hospital Association, 1975.

Parker, Luther R. "Collective Bargaining in Pharmacy?" American Journal of Hospital Pharmacy 27 (March 1970): 209-12.

Phillips, D. F. "Cook County Hospital: Politics and Power Plays." Hospitals 50 (March 16, 1976): 101-3.

Pointer, Dennis D. "Catholic Hospitals' Dual Nature Complicates Labor Relations Strategy." Hospital Progress 57 (February 1976): 58.

_____. Unionization, Collective Bargaining and the Non-Profit Hospital. College of Business Administration, Center for Labor and Management Monograph Series no. 13. Iowa City: University of Iowa, 1969.

Provost, George P. "Collective Bargaining through Affiliated Chapters ?" American Journal of Hospital Pharmacy 27 (March 1970): 187.

"Quality Not Negotiable." Hospitals 48 (October 16, 1974): 43.

"Racial Discrimination and Collective Bargaining." Newsletter of the American Society of Hospital Attorneys 6 (April 1973): 5.

Robinson, A. S. "Collective Bargaining in the Technical and Professional Field." Personnel Journal 55 (June 1976): 278-81.

Rosasco, Louise C. "Collective Bargaining: What's a Director of Nursing to Do?" Hospitals 48 (September 15, 1974): 79-80.

Rosmann, Joseph. "Hospital Revenue Controls—Their Labor Relations and Labor Force Utilization Implications for the Hospital

Industry." Paper presented to the Thirtieth National Conference on Labor, May 17, 1977, at New York University.

_____. "Implications of Third-Party Cost Control Efforts for the Collective Bargaining Process in the Hospital Industry." Unpublished paper. Chicago: American Hospital Association, n.d.

Rotham, William A., and William A. Himmelsbach, Jr. "Study of Michigan Contracts in Michigan Indicates That There Is a Wide Variety of Provisions in Such Documents." Hospitals 45 (December 16, 1971): 67-71.

Rutsohn, P. D., and R. M. Grimes. "Nightingaleism and Negotiation—New Attitudes of Health Professionals." Personnel Journal 56 (August 1977): 398-401.

Sammons, James H. "American Medical Association Explains Negotiations Department." Hospitals 50 (May 16, 1976): 113.

Sargis, Mary. "Collective Bargaining in the Nursing Profession: The Hospital 'Director' as Object of Special Study." Ed.D. dissertation, Columbia University Teachers College, 1977.

Saxton, Dolores F. "Collective Bargaining in Academe: A Personal Appraisal." Nursing Outlook 21 (November 1973): 704-7.

Schramm, Carl J. "Containing Hospital Labor Costs—A Separate-Industries Approach." Employee Relations Law Journal 4 (Summer 1978): 82-97.

Seidman, Joel. "Nurses and Collective Bargaining." Industrial and Labor Relations Review 23 (April 1970): 335-51.

Semeraro, Richard A. "Collective Bargaining in Voluntary Non-profit Institutions—The Management View as Seen in Universities and Hospitals." In Collective Bargaining Today: Proceedings of the Collective Bargaining Forum, 1970, Institute of Collective Bargaining and Group Relations, pp. 260-68. Washington, D.C.: Bureau of National Affairs, 1971.

Singleton, B. W. "Negotiating a Collective Bargaining Agreement." Hospital Progress 56 (October 1975): 57.

Spirn, Steven. "Negotiating and Coexisting with a Union." Hospital Progress 57 (February 1976): 54-55.

Steele, Mark M. "AMA Teaches Physicians to Fight Back." Modern Health Care 6 (July 1976): 31.

Steve, Laurence. "Labor Negotiations and the Director of Physical Therapy." Physical Therapy 53 (June 1973): 623-27.

Swanberg, Gloria. "Nursing/Labor Negotiating." Hospitals 44 (August 1, 1970): 54-56.

"Union Teams up with Black Power." Business Week, April 15, 1969, pp. 22-24.

"Unions Decide." Hospital and Health Services Review 70 (August 1974): 263-65.

Van Cleve, William J. "Collective Bargaining in the Health Care Industry." Journal of the American Dietetic Association 61 (December 1972): 633-36.

Vittetoe, Marie C. "Exploratory Study of Collective Bargaining Contracts Covering Medical Technologists." Ph.D. dissertation, West Virginia University, 1973.

Vladeck, Judith. "Collective Bargaining in Voluntary Hospitals and Other Nonprofit Operations." In Proceedings of New York University Nineteenth Annual Conference on Labor, edited by Thomas G. S. Christensen, pp. 221-33. Washington, D.C.: Bureau of National Affairs, 1967.

Weatherbee, Robert A. Nurses and Collective Bargaining in the Bay Area. Berkeley: University of California, 1968.

Werther, W. B., Jr., et al. "Collective Action and Cooperation in the Health Professions." Journal of Nursing Administration 7 (July-August 1977): 13-19.

Yager, Paul. "The Mediators' Dilemma." Paper presented at the Thirtieth National Conference on Labor, May 17, 1977, at New York University.

Zimmerman, Anne. "American Nurses' Association Economic Security Program in Retrospect." Nursing Forum 10 (1971): 312-21.

Contract Administration

Alper, Philip R., ed. Doctors' Unions and Collective Bargaining: Report of a Proceedings Conference of the Institute of Industrial Relations and American Federation of Physicians and Dentists, 1974, at the University of California at Berkeley.

"ANA's Economic and General Welfare Program: The Grievance Procedure." American Nursing Association Publication EC-132 (1975): 1-16.

Amundson, Norman E. "Labor Relations and the Nursing Leader (Past Practice Is Killing Us!)." Journal of Nursing Administration 3 (November-December 1973): 12-13.

Bennett, Richard, and Ruth M. MacRobert. "Building Skills in Disciplining and Grievance Handling." Hospital Topics (January-February 1975): 8, and (March-April 1975): 50-55.

Camerano, Franklin. "Grievance Procedure, Heart of Collective Bargaining Agreement." Hospital Topics 43 (August 1965): 49-54.

Cleland, Virginia S. "The Supervisor in Collective Bargaining." Journal of Nursing Administration 4 (1975): 33-35.

Clelland, Rod. "Grievance Procedures: Outlet for Employee, Insight for Management." In Hospital Organization and Management, edited by Jonathan S. Rakich, pp. 269-72. St. Louis: Catholic Hospital Association, 1972.

Connor, P. J. "Unions Are Here—Here's How to Cope." Modern Hospital 107 (August 1966): 102-4.

Elkin, Randyl D. "Negotiating and Administrating a Union Contract." Hospital Progress 56 (January 1975): 40-43.

Fleishman, Raymond. "Living with a Contract." Hospitals 47 (November 16, 1973): 51-54.

Gregorich, P., et al. "Experts Exchange Views on Grievance Procedures in Hospitals." Hospitals 52 (August 16, 1978): 68-73.

Gronbach, R. C. "Three-Step Grievance Procedure." Hospitals 37 (January 16, 1963): 60-62.

Hahn, J. E., et al. "Employees Reinforce This Grievance Plan." Modern Hospital 103 (November 1964): 99-101.

Horty, John F. "Do Contracts Say What They Mean?" Hospitals 50 (April 1, 1976): 72.

Howard, David L. "Views on A.S.H.P.'s Involvement in Collective Bargaining." American Journal of Hospital Pharmacy 27 (March 1970): 217-20.

Juris, Hervey, Joseph Rosmann, Charles Maxey, and Gail Bentivegna. "Employees Discipline No Longer Management Prerogative Only." Hospitals 51 (May 1, 1977): 67-68.

Larkins, Eddie L. "Study of Grievances, 1971-1973, University Hospital, Ann Arbor, Michigan." Master's thesis, University of Michigan, 1974.

Mauksch, Ingeborg G. "Attainment of Control over Professional Practice." Nursing Forum 10 (1971): 232-38.

Metzger, Norman. "Living with a Collective Bargaining Agreement the First 100 Days." Hospital Management 98 (October 1964): 49-52.

_____. "Voluntary Arbitration on Contract Administration Disputes." Hospital Progress 51 (September 1970): 48-51.

Natonski, J. "Why a Union Contract Didn't Work at Our Hospital . . . Midland (Michigan) Hospital Center." RN 41 (May 1978): 69-71.

Norville, J., and R. J. Halonen. "Negotiating and Administering Contracts with Hospital-Based Physicians." Hospital Progress 56 (June 1975): 61-67.

Spirn, S. "Negotiating and Coexisting with a Union." Hospital Progress 57 (February 1976): 54-55.

Vittetoe, Marie C. "Exploratory Study of Collective Bargaining Contracts Covering Medical Technologists." Ph.D. dissertation, West Virginia University, 1973.

Wynne, D. "A Union Contract Was the Only Language Our Hospital Would Understand." RN 41 (May 1978): 66-68.

Disputes

Extent, Form, and Location

Aboud, Antone, and Grace Sterrett Aboud. Rights to Strike in Public Employment. Ithaca, N.Y.: Cornell University, New York State School of Industrial and Labor Relations, 1974.

Anderson, Arvid. Compulsory Arbitration in Public Sector Dispute Settlement—An Alternative View. Dispute Settlement in the Public Sector Research Series, vol. 1. Iowa City: University of Iowa, Center for Labor Management, 1972.

Badgley, R. F. "Health Worker Strikes: Social and Economic Bases of Conflict." International Journal of Health Services 5 (1975): 9-17.

"Bargaining—Yes, Strike—No. Plan Has ANA Endorsement." American Journal of Nursing 70 (February 1970): 222.

Barrett, Jerome T., and Ira B. Lobel. "Public Sector Strikes—Legislative and Court Treatment." Monthly Labor Review 97 (September 1974): 19-22.

Bennett, Richard, and Ruth M. MacRobert. "Building Skills in Disciplining and Grievance Handling." Hospital Topics (January-February 1975): 8, and (March-April 1975): 50-55.

Berkeley, A. Eliot, ed. Labor Relations in Hospitals and Health Care Facilities: Proceedings of a Conference Presented by the American Arbitration Association and the Federal Conciliation Service. Washington, D.C.: Bureau of National Affairs, 1976.

Berman, J. D. "Strikes by House Staff." Journal of the American Medical Association 240 (August 25, 1978): 736.

Bullough, Bonnie. "The New Militancy in Nursing." Nursing Forum 10 (1971): 273-88.

Carlton, D. R. "Views from Both Sides of the Picket Line." Modern Hospital 104 (June 1965): 76-79.

"Charleston Blues." Economist 231 (May 3, 1969): 47-48.

Cleary, D. M. "A Nonstrike for Patient Care." Modern Health Care 3 (June 1975): 43-44.

Cuming, M. W. "Industrial Action: A Note on Administrative Practice during the Action by Hospital Ancillary Staff, Spring 1973." Hospital and Health Services Review 70 (April 1974): 122-24.

Cunningham, R. M., Jr. "Strike." Modern Health Care 5 (February 1976): 41-48.

"Doctor's Strike: Peace with Promises." Medical World News 14 (April 6, 1973): 8.

Ecenbarger, William. "Second Thoughts about the Right to Strike." Private Practice 5 (July 1973): 36-37.

Hacker, John S. "Militant Actions by Nurses in Collective Bargaining in Voluntary Not-for-Profit Hospitals: An Exploratory Analysis." Master's thesis, University of Iowa, 1973.

Hart, Harold H. Strike: For and against Introduction. New York: Hart, 1971.

Hill, S. G. "The Right to Strike." The Hospital 67 (May 1971): 151-54.

Hobart, C. L. "Collective Bargaining with Professionals: Conflict, Containment, or Accommodation?" Health Care Management Review 1 (Spring 1976): 7-16.

Jarvis, P. "Nursing and the Ethics of Withdrawing Professional Services." Nursing Mirror 146 (February 16, 1978): 30-31.

"Lay Interference Spawns Union and Strike." Medical World News 14 (February 16, 1973): 18-19.

"Make 'em Shoot Us: Strike!" Oklahoma State Medical Association Journal 65 (July 1972): 247.

"Maryland Association Recognizes Pharmacist's Union, and May Step into Disputes with Owners." American Druggist 165 (March 6, 1972): 41.

Match, Robert K., et al. "Unionization Strikes, Threatened Strikes, and Hospitals—The View from Hospital Management." International Journal of Health Services 5 (1975): 27-36.

McGregor, Maurice. "Strike and Physician." Canadian Medical Association Journal 105 (December 1971): 1139-41.

McVeigh, Robert C. "Confrontation." Prism 1 (August 1973): 22-25.

Meilicke, Carl A. "Saskatchewan Medical Care Dispute of 1962: An Analytical Social History." Ph.D. dissertation, University of Minnesota, 1967.

Miller, Michael H. "Nurses' Right to Strike." Journal of Nursing Administration 5 (February 1975): 35-39.

"Monsignor Envisions 'no contract, no work' as New Religious Vows." RN 37 (September 1974): 36.

Mueller, William J. "Dangers of Direct ASHP Involvement in Collective Bargaining." American Journal of Hospital Pharmacy 27 (March 1970): 213-16.

Nash, Al. "Labor-Management Conflict and Change in a Hospital." Hospital Administration 21 (1976): 44-63.

_____. "Labor-Management Conflict in a Voluntary Hospital." Ph.D. dissertation, New York University, 1972.

"Obligatory Triad: The Conflict in Hospital Administration." Personnel Journal 47 (August 1968): 582-84.

"Physicians Unionize to Fight 'Third-Party Interference'." Hospitals 46 (June 16, 1972): 118.

Pointer, Dennis D., and Harry E. Graham. "Recognition, Negotiations and Work Stoppages in Hospitals." Monthly Labor Review 94 (May 1971): 54-58.

Pointer, Dennis D., and Norman Metzger. "Work Stoppages in the Hospital Industry: A Preliminary Profile and Analysis." Hospital Administration 17 (Spring 1972): 9-24.

Reed, E. A. "Do Strikes in Hospitals Justify Goals?" American Operating Room Nurses Journal 22 (July 1975): 27-28.

"Revolt of the Hospital Workers." Ebony, March 1971, pp. 53-58.

Scheiber, I. B. "Report on Labor Dispute: Public Health Nurse Association and the City of New York." Labor Law Journal 17 (July 1966): 401-12.

Schrader, Elinor S. "Supervisory Nurses Caught in Increasing Tensions." Association of Operating Room Nurses Journal 21 (February 1975): 191-92.

Schulz, Rockwell, and Alton C. Johnson. "Conflict in Hospitals." Hospital Administration 16 (Summer 1971): 36-50.

"Strike Actions Termed Emergency Measures." American Druggist 161 (June 29, 1970): 22.

Stukalin, R. L. "A Case Study of the Contingency Planning Process of a Major Medical Center Preparing for an Employee Strike." MBA thesis, City University of New York, Baruch College, 1973.

Taft, Robert. "A Right to Expect Continuous Health Care Services." Texas Hospitals 29 (January 1974): 17.

Tuck, J. N. "The Question for AMA: When Is a Strike Not a Strike?" Modern Health Care 4 (August 1975): 160.

Veatch, R. M. "Interns and Residents on Strike." Inquiry 5 (December 1975): 7-8.

Wolfe, S. "Worker Conflicts in the Health Field: An Overview." International Journal of Health Services 5 (1975): 5-8.

Impact

Appelbaum, Alan L. "The Meaning of the New York Strike." Hospitals 49 (April 6, 1975): 17a.

"Binding Up Wounds in a Hospital Strike." Business Week, June 14, 1969, p. 54.

Brody, Paul E., and Jordan London. "How Costly Is a Strike?" Hospitals 49 (September 16, 1975): 53-56.

Cameron, John. "Strike Weapon." Nursing Mirror 130 (February 27, 1970): 10.

Coulton, M. R. "Labor Disputes: A Challenge to Nurse Staffing." Journal of Nursing Administration 6 (May 1976): 15-20.

"First Results of Doctor Strikes Include Backlash." Medical World News 16 (June 30, 1975): 16-19.

Fishbein, Morris. "On Man's Inhumanity to Man." Medical World News 14 (December 14, 1973): 92.

Folker, David A., and S. D. Pomrinse. "Preparations for Potential Strike." Hospitals 47 (September 16, 1973): 51-55.

Fuchs, Sheldon. "Planning for a Hospital Strike." Health Care Engineering 2 (July-August 1974): 28-30.

Hacker, John S. "Militant Actions by Nurses in Collective Bargaining in Voluntary Not-for-Profit Hospitals: An Exploratory Analysis." Master's thesis, University of Iowa, 1973.

Hickox, Robert F. "Can You Win Out in a Walkout?" Hospital World 1 (July 1972): 7-10.

Hiscock, H. H. "County Medical Societies Should Develop Plans to Handle Future Hospital Strikes." Michigan Medicine 69 (December 1970): 1061.

Hobart, C. L. "Collective Bargaining with Professionals: Conflict, Containment, or Accommodation?" Health Care Management Review 1 (Spring 1976): 7-16.

Hogben, George L., and Robert Shulman. "Patient and Staff Reactions to a Strike by Essential Hospital Employees." American Journal of Psychiatry 133 (December 1976): 1464-65.

Kennedy, Alan. "California Hospital Fight—Round Two." Medical World News 14 (March 23, 1973): 4.

"Laundries and Catering Hit by Ancillary Workers' Strike." Nursing Times 69 (March 8, 1973): 296-97.

Lihach, Nadine. "San Francisco: Winners and Losers." Modern Health Care 2 (October 1974): 32-34.

McGregor, Maurice. "Strike and Physician." Canadian Medical Association Journal 105 (December 1971): 1139-41.

McVeigh, Robert C. "Confrontation." Prism 1 (August 1973): 22-25.

Metzger, Norman. "Hospital Industry Challenged to Develop via Unified Approach When Union Negotiations Break Down." Hospital Management 111 (June 1971): 1.

"New York's House Staff Strike." Hospital Practice 10 (June 1975): 143-52.

Reaves, J. L. "Decisions to Strike." Journal of Practical Nursing 26 (June 1976): 25.

Roach, David L., et al. "Hospitals Stand Firm, Ensure Care in Lengthy, Area-Wide Nurses' Strike." Hospitals 51 (August 1, 1977): 49-51.

Ross, B. T. "Computerized System Aids Staffing in Strikes." Hospitals 50 (September 16, 1975): 49-52.

Schorr, Thelma M. "They'd Better Believe." American Journal of Nursing 74 (August 1974): 1415.

Schreiber, I. B. "Report on Labor Dispute: Public Health Nurse Association and the City of New York." Labor Law Journal 17 (July 1966): 401-12.

Schwartz, Harry. "Public Will Not Tolerate Disruptive Strikes." Hospitals 49 (November 16, 1975): 43-46.

Smith, David A. "Strike! Or—Why Not to Join a Union." Pennsylvania Medicine 76 (January 1973): 33.

Spencer, Vernon, et al. "One Strike . . . and You're Apt to Be Out." Hospital Management 101 (March 1966): 34-41.

"Strike Closes 10 Revco Prescription Departments." American Druggist 160 (December 1, 1969): 21.

Stukalin, R. L. "A Case Study of the Contingency Planning Process of a Major Medical Center Preparing for an Employee Strike." MBA thesis, City University of New York, Baruch College, 1973.

Wood, J. F., et al. "Mandate for Strike Actions." Nursing Mirror 139 (August 30, 1974): 34-35.

Dispute Resolution

Mechanisms: Arbitration, Mediation,
and Fact Finding

"American Society for Medical Technology Positions Statement on
Collective Bargaining and Position Definitions." American Journal of Medical Technologists 42 (May 8, 1976): 42.

Amundson, Norman E. "Labor Relations and the Nursing Leader
(Alternatives to the Strike in Collective Bargaining." Journal of
Nursing Administration 5 (January 1975): 11-12.

_____. "Labor Relations and the Nursing Leader (Labor Arbitra-
tion)." Journal of Nursing Administration 4 (March-April 1974):
16-17.

Anderson, Arvid. Compulsory Arbitration in Public Sector Dispute
Settlement—An Alternative View. Dispute Settlement in the Pub-
lic Sector Research Series, vol. 1. Iowa City: University of
Iowa, Center for Labor Management, 1972.

Baderschneider, Earl R., and Paul F. Miller, eds. Labor Arbitration in Health Care: A Case Book. Health Systems Management
Series. New York: Halsted Press, 1976.

Benjamin, H. E. "Collective Bargaining and the Hospitals." Unpublished paper, Princeton University, Industrial Relations Section, 1969.

Berkeley, A. Eliot, ed. Labor Relations in Hospitals and Health
Care Facilities: Proceedings of a Conference Presented by the
American Arbitration Association and the Federal Conciliation
Service. Washington, D.C.: Bureau of National Affairs, 1976.

Campbell, Michael. "Solving Union Negotiation Problems." Executive Housekeeper 20 (October 1973): 38-41.

Coulton, M. R. "Labor Disputes: A Challenge to Nurse Staffing."
Journal of Nursing Administration 6 (May 1976): 15-20.

Denton, J. A. "Attitudes toward Alternative Models of Unions and
Professional Associations." Nurse Resident 25 (May-June 1976):
178-80.

"Dispute Resolution through AAA and NCDS Services: 'Preventative Medicine' in the Health Care Field." Arbitration News, February 1973, pp. 1-5.

Dunlap, Karen. "Mediation—Arbitration: Reactions from Rank and File." Monthly Labor Review 96 (September 1973): 65-66.

Greaves, F. "How to Create a Strike Contingency Plan." Medical Laboratory Observer 9 (April 1977): 73.

Herndon, Robert E. "Arbitration: How to Go About It." Personnel 47 (May-June 1970): 24-28.

Hines, R. J. "Mandatory Contract Arbitration—Is It a Viable Process?" Industrial and Labor Relations Review 25 (July 1972): 533-44.

Kagel, Sam. "Combining Mediation and Arbitration." Monthly Labor Review 96 (September 1973): 62-63.

Kessler, Harold D. "Guidelines for Resolving Labor Disputes." Hospital Progress 51 (September 1970): 52-55.

Kheel, Theodore W., and Lewis B. Kaden. "Collective Bargaining in Hospitals: A Plan to Resolve Impasses." In Proceedings of the Twenty-Second Annual Winter Meeting of the Industrial Relations Research Association, edited by Gerald G. Somers, pp. 210-16. Madison: Industrial Relations Research Association, 1970.

Kheel, Theodore W., and Lewis B. Kaden. "Plan to Resolve Impasses in Hospital Bargaining." Monthly Labor Review 93 (April 1970): 45-48.

Metzger, Norman. "Arbitration Procedure." Hospitals 48 (April 16, 1974): 47-49, and (May 1, 1974): 45-47.

_____. "Hospital Industry Challenged to Develop via Unified Approach When Union Negotiations Break Down." Hospital Management 111 (June 1971): 1.

Miller, P. A. A Study to Investigate the Effect of Compulsory Arbitration Legislation on the Collective Bargaining Process. Abstracts of Hospital Management Studies, vol. 9, no. 1. Toronto: University of Ottawa, 1973.

Polland, Harry. "Mediation—Arbitration: A Trade Union View."
Monthly Labor Review 96 (September 1973): 63-65.

Rimer, J. Thomas. "Arbitration: How to Avoid It." Personnel
47 (May-June 1970): 29-33.

Rogan, Peter G. "Private Non-Profit Hospitals: A Viable Alternative to the Strike." Hospital Administration 19 (Spring 1974):
22-55.

Sabghir, Irving H. "Some Reflections on Mediation, Factfinding
and Arbitration in the Health Care Industry." Paper presented
at the Third Annual Meeting, Society of Professionals in Dispute
Resolution, Los Angeles, October 13, 1975.

Scearce, J. F., and L. D. Tanner. "Health Care Bargaining: The
FMCS Experience." Labor Law Journal 27 (July 1976): 387-98.

Van Asselt, K. A. "Collective Bargaining in the Public Services:
Impasse Resolution Procedures." Public Administration Review
32 (March-April 1972): 114-19.

Wolfe, S. "Worker Conflicts in the Health Field: An Overview."
International Journal of Health Services 5 (1975): 5-8.

Success

Baderschneider, Earl R., and Paul F. Miller, eds. Labor Arbitration in Health Care: A Case Book. Health Systems Management
Series. New York: Halsted Press, 1976.

"Binding up Wounds in a Hospital Strike." Business Week, June 14,
1969, p. 54.

Chandrasekharan, K. An Exploration of a Viable Process of Collective Bargaining in Nonprofit Hospitals Minimizing the Strike Potential. Knoxville: University of Tennessee.

DiPaolo, V. "84-Day Strike Ends in Youngstown." Modern Health
Care 8 (March 1978): 24.

"Dispute Resolution through AAA and NCDS Services: 'Preventative
Medicine' in the Health Care Field." Arbitration News, February 1973, pp. 1-5.

Gamble, Stephen W. "Coping with a Strike by Doctors." Hospitals 50 (September 1, 1976): 61-64.

Hickox, Robert F. "Can You Win Out in a Walkout?" Hospital World 1 (July 1972): 7-10.

Hines, R. J. "Mandatory Contract Arbitration—Is It a Viable Process?" Industrial and Labor Relations Review 25 (July 1972): 533-44.

Hobart, C. L. "Collective Bargaining with Professionals: Conflict, Containment, or Accommodation?" Health Care Management Review 1 (Spring 1976): 7-16.

Metzger, Norman. "Compulsory Arbitration Stifles Negotiations." Hospital Progress 51 (May 1970): 96.

Reed, E. A. "Do Strikes in Hospitals Justify Goals?" American Operating Room Nurses Journal 22 (July 1975): 27-28.

"Revco Settles Strike but Bypasses Society." American Druggist 160 (December 15, 1969): 16.

Ross, B. T. "Computerized System Aids Staffing in Strikes." Hospitals 50 (September 16, 1975): 50-52.

INTERNATIONAL AND COMPARATIVE
HOSPITAL LABOR RELATIONS

Abbis, C. "The Quebec Hospital Strike." Canadian Hospital 43 (August 1966): 20A-20B.

Bradford, J. D. "B.C. Hospitals Learn to Live with Labor." Canadian Hospitals 52 (January 1965): 33-35.

Cormick, Gerald W. "The Collective Bargaining Experience of Canadian Registered Nurses." Labor Law Journal 20 (October 1969): 667-82.

Derraugh, W. K. "Union and Personnel Relations." Canadian Hospitals 40 (November 1963): 54-55.

Employment and Conditions of Work and Life of Nursing Personnel. Report 7, Part 2, Sixty-first Session of the International Labour Conference, 1976.

Gilchrist, J., ed. "Perspective." Canadian Nurse 73 (May 1977): 3.

Giovannetti, R. J. "What Groups of Employees Will the Union Attempt to Organize?" Journal of the American Health Care Association 3 (July 1977): 5.

Gould, D. "Breakfast in Bed?" Nursing Times 73 (January 27, 1977): 116.

Grandre, L. de. "American Medical Unionism: Does Patient or Third Party Retain the Doctor?" Canadian Medical Association Journal 109 (October 20, 1973): 800.

Grant, R. A. "Impact of the Supervisor on the Collective Agreement." Canadian Hospitals 49 (October 1972): 29.

_____. "Unions Exist Because of Management's Short-Sightedness." Canadian Hospitals 50 (January 1973): 8.

Heller, T. "Nurses Unite." Nursing Times 73 (May 5, 1977): 640-41.

Inglis, Margaret. Collective Bargaining and the Nurses: A Study of Selected Aspects of Collective Bargaining by Graduate Nurses in the Public General Hospitals of the Province of Ontario. Toronto: University of Toronto, 1969.

"Interns in B.C. Sign First Agreement." Labor Gazette 77 (June 1977): 242.

"Interview: David Williams." Nursing Times 73 (October 27, 1977): 1661.

Hones, E. "Accepting the Trade Union Role." Midwives Chronicle 90 (September 1977): 206.

LeBourdais, Isabel. "Collective Bargaining: R.N.A.O." Canadian Nurse 61 (July 1965): 529-32.

Lewis, S. S. "Nurses and Trade Unions in Britain." International Journal of Health Services 6 (1976): 641-49.

Little, Stanley A. "Hospitals and Unions." Canadian Hospitals 43 (March 1966): 50.

Maeken, J. J. "21st Annual Industrial Relations Conference. Theme: Industrial Relations and Economic Management." LAMP 34 (December 1977): 9–13.

MacRury, A. "Handling Management-Labor Disputes in Hospitals." Hospital Administration in Canada 16 (August 1974): 35–36.

Meeks, J. R. "Unions and Management Join to Educate Supervisors." Dimensions of Health Service 54 (July 1977): 41–42.

Moga, Michael D. The Impact of Joint or Multi-Employer Bargaining on Hospital Labour Relations in Ontario. Toronto: University of Toronto, 1972.

Morgan, Dorothy M. "Role of the Director of Nursing in Collective Bargaining." Canadian Hospitals 50 (January 1973): 44.

"Negotiated Wages and Working Conditions in Ontario Hospitals, March 1970." Toronto: Ontario Department of Labour, 1970.

"Provisions in Major Collective Agreements in Canadian Hospitals." Labor Gazette 71 (December 1971): 792–95.

Riches, L. N. "Trade Practices Act Proposed Amendments— Vicious Attack on Unions and Unionists." Royal Australian Nursing Federation Review 8 (May 1977): 4.

Rowe, G. A. "Handling Hospital Labor Relations." Hospital Administration in Canada 12 (July 1970): 46–50.

Spanswick, A. "Why Nurses Should Join a Trade Union." Nursing Mirror 143 (September 9, 1976): 39–40.

"The Way Ahead." Nursing Times 72 (December 2, 1976): 1857.

Watkin, B. "Independent Trade Union No. 510T." Nursing Mirror 144 (June 30, 1977): 10.

_____. "Join 'em and Beat 'em." Nursing Mirror 143 (September 9, 1976): 41.

_____. "Rule of Law." Nursing Mirror 144 (May 5, 1977): 42.

"What Is the TUC?" Nursing Times 73 (May 12, 1977): 684–85.

Wigham, E. "Nursing: A Suitable Profession for Treatment." LAMP 33 (October 1976): 5.

Wilson, Donald C. E. An Analysis of the Approach by Hospitals in Ontario to Collective Bargaining. Toronto: School of Hygiene, Department of Hospital Administration, University of Toronto, June 1966.